pamela smith's
healthy living
cookbook

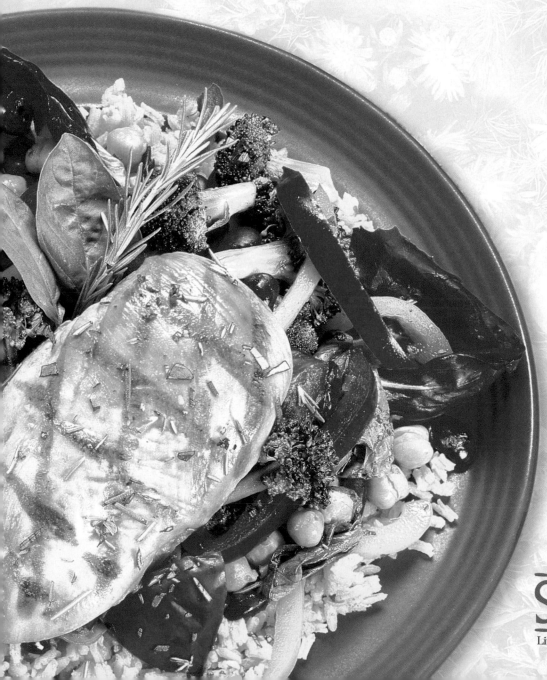

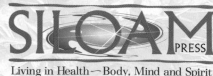
SILOAM PRESS

Living in Health—Body, Mind and Spirit

PAMELA SMITH'S HEALTHY LIVING COOKBOOK by Pamela Smith
Published by Siloam Press
A part of Strang Communications Company
600 Rinehart Road
Lake Mary, FL 32746
www.siloampress.com

Unless otherwise noted, all Scripture quotations are from the Holy Bible, New International Version. Copyright © 1973, 1978, 1984, International Bible Society. Used by permission.

Meal pictured on cover: Chicken Marco (pg. 114)

Cover design: Pat Theriault
Interior design: Pat Theriault
Typography: Jeanne Logue
Photography: Debi Harbin

Library of Congress Catalog Card Number: 2001098056
International Standard Book Number: 0-88419-787-5

Portions of this book were previously published as *The Good Life*, copyright © 1995 by Creation House, ISBN 0-88419-400-0.

02 03 04 05 06 07 — 9 8 7 6 5 4 3 2 1
Printed in the United States of America

quest for healthy living

Greetings! So much has happened in the world—and in the world of food—in the seven years since I first wrote *The Good Life.* Yet, joyfully, so much has remained the same.

Science continues to reveal the power of good food to get us well and keep us well—showing us the basic recipe for healthy living. The same principles of what it takes to live well apply as much today as they did in 1995.

Many of those medical revelations have had an impact on what we find in the grocery store and in restaurants. It's no longer a major hunt to find whole-grain pastas or brown rice, and there is now a vast array of quality produce and foods from which to choose. The extremely talented chefs we read about and see on TV are using their classical training to create bold-flavored dishes that are healthier for us—and have brought many once-foreign tastes and techniques into our everyday kitchens and restaurants. I am so very grateful to the many chefs I work with who daily introduce me to extraordinary tastes, flavors, textures and presentations—and to my travels that have increased my own repertoire of ingredients and cooking techniques. I now pull recipe inspiration from cultures around the world—Mediterranean, Latin, Asian, Provencal—and that is reflected in my pantry and meal planning. The basics of great cooking have been enhanced even more—resulting in meals that are fresh, elegant and uncomplicated.

However, life has gotten even more busy—even more time-pushed and demanding—not only for myself but seemingly for the world in general. My clients, readers and the visitors to my website have raised a loud cry to make living well even more simple and healthy recipes even more quick and easy to prepare. And that is what this book is all about—taking the "right stuff" of *The Good Life*—and adding in more tips and helps to make it a simple, quick and delicious guide to cooking for healthy living.

I am encouraged that there is still so much to learn, to adapt and to discover that can help us in our ever-growing quest for healthy living. I do hope that you enjoy these recipes—and that this guide will become an often referred to essential in your kitchen—and a trusted vehicle for living well.

Blessings!
Pam

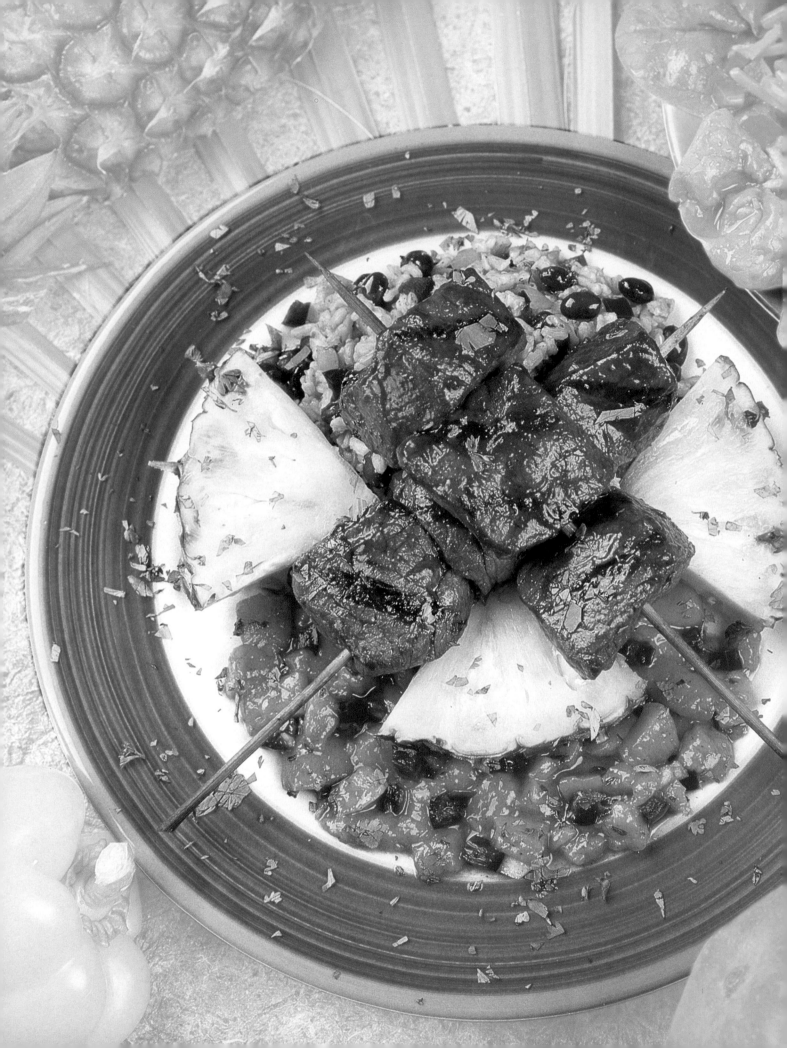

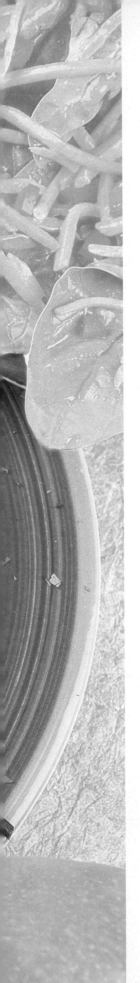

contents

Beef Tip Skewers (pg. 129)

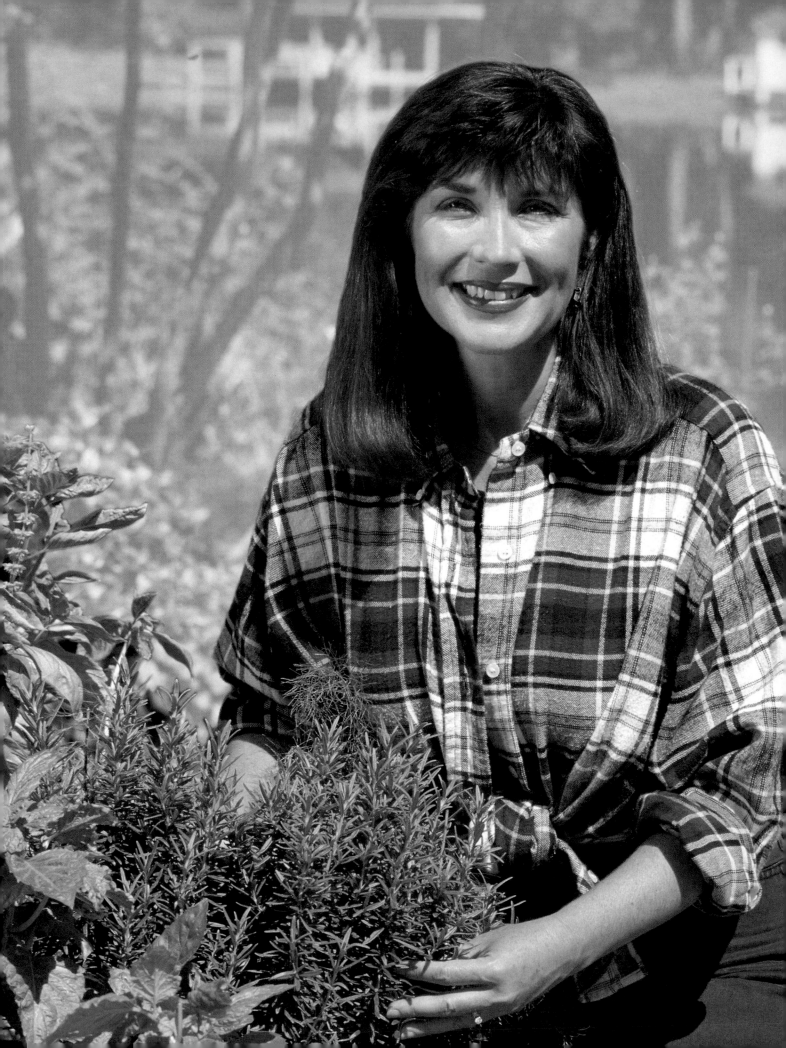

make it healthy; make it quick

Food, and the sharing of food, sustains human relationships. It's an extraordinarily important part of the family structure, and it's the common denominator that brings people together in the house.

Cooking and eating good food is a great life pleasure—and there's nothing wrong with that—except that for too long, good often meant "unhealthy" and sure to be loaded with excess fats, sugars and salt. Healthy has been construed to be bland, boring and tasteless.

However, contrary to what many people have experienced, healthy food can—and should—be colorful, delicious and quick and easy to prepare. For food to be enjoyable, it needs to taste great. If it doesn't taste good, it has limited power to satisfy.

Healthy living cooking and dining is guided by the premise that good health and good food are synonymous. It's an approach to food

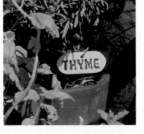

preparation and presentation that serves up meals that delight and nourish. This kind of cooking makes eating what we like the same as eating what is good for us. The food is fresh and flavorful, relying on herbs, garlic, fresh vegetables, fruits and small amounts of high-quality olive oil. No rich sauces, heavy starches or fats to dull the senses. Meals consist of carefully selected dishes served in appropriate portions.

Each dish in this *Healthy Living Cookbook* is created from natural, wholesome foods that are high in natural fiber and nutrients. The meals are designed to be low in fat and calories, low in cholesterol and sodium, but high on flavor and beauty. And one more thing: They are

Pictured: Pam Smith

make it healthy; make it quick

designed for those of us who don't have the time (or often the energy) to plan and cook a meal after a busy day.

Let's face it: Time is short. Often we are mentally and emotionally exhausted from the thousand-and-one demands of living life in this twenty-first century. On weeknights especially, spending less time in the kitchen becomes a clear necessity if we are to spend more time enjoying our family, friends and our food. Too often, in our catch-as-catch-can way of doing things, something is compromised—taste, health or the entire satisfaction and fulfillment of making and enjoying a home-cooked meal.

Today's supermarkets carry a wide range of healthy and tasty foods that have opened the door to meals that are much more interesting and can be made in quick order. The recipes in this cookbook are personal ones I want to share with you to help you overcome the obstacles to healthy cooking. They are the quickest and easiest ways to turn simple recipes into elegant, complete meals—both for everyday and for special occasions. These meals won't leave you or your guest feeling deprived of the finer things in life. I have chosen the recipes for ease, speed and flavor. I have chosen my meals and presentations for fun and enjoyment.

With that said, I also believe that a major part of healthy living is not to spend any unnecessary time in the kitchen! My theory about cooking has always been, "If it takes longer to cook it than to eat it, FORGET IT!" How about you?

In the next section you will find some basic pointers to "make it quick!" Try them out; you'll be glad you did.

Cooking-Quick Survival Tips

- Keep your pantry, fridge and freezer well-stocked with the basic ingredients for quick and easy food preparation. (See "The Well-Stocked Kitchen," pages 34–47.)

- Keep an ongoing grocery list, and jot down items as soon as you begin to run low. If you wait until you are completely out of an item, it could cost you an unplanned trip to the store.

- Since half the battle is just deciding what to prepare, one or two days in advance, pick out the meal you are going to try—and make sure you have the needed ingredients on hand. If you have a family, enlist them in this time of preparing—even assigning them the responsibility of a meal or two each week.

- Usually a recipe takes longer the first time you prepare it, so when you plan to make a new dish, give yourself the extra edge of time.

- If an entrée requires a bit more time to prepare, put it together with a simpler side dish. These *Healthy Living* menus are designed so that your time and effort may be spent on one part of the meal.

Keep a Ready-to-Cook Kitchen

- Do most of your food preparation on a countertop close to your sink.

- De-clutter your countertops by storing your seldom-used appliances in less-accessible cabinets.

- Use the drawer and cabinet closest to your cooking area to store knives, vegetable scrub brushes and peelers, stirring spoons, measuring spoons and cups, mixing bowls, colanders, cutting boards, scales and graters.

- Keep your food processor and hand-held blender close so they are always handy for quick chopping, mincing or blending.

The Clock Is Ticking!

You'll find a time clock at the heading of specially selected recipes that can be prepared in less than thirty minutes—and even less if you have items pre-prepped and ready to fire. That is the secret of quick cooking. All professional kitchens employ a technique called *mise en place*, which means organizing and pre-prepping your ingredients so that you are ready to cook. It does wonders for speeding up your cooking time, keeping your sanity and assuring a dish without forgotten ingredients.

Time is such an issue that even if you're fired up with the ambition to cook healthy, great-tasting meals, you still have to consider how much time you have to shop and cook. Begin by taking stock of what you're doing now for breakfast, lunch and dinner. Try tackling just one of the day's meals at a time. Which would you like to change first?

For breakfast, you might like to find some simple everyday alternatives to cereal or a bagel—or no breakfast at all. All the breakfasts can be made in less than thirty minutes—even the muffins can be made in advance and frozen for a quick pop-out. The Country French Toast is simple and quick to make on order, but you can speed up the process even more by having pre-grilled slices frozen and ready to pop in the toaster. Making the Homemade Pancake Mix in abundance and storing it in the refrigerator allows you to make pancakes in a hurry.

Of course, some breakfasts can be put together with minimal fuss or effort—and in less than five minutes! These are:

- Granola Breakfast (page 68)
- Whole-Grain Cereal With Berries (page 68)
- Freshly Fruited Yogurt Parfait (page 69)
- Fresh Fruit Shake (page 69)
- Cinnamon Raisin Oatmeal (page 71)
- Nicole's Cheesy Hash Browns (page 71)
- Garden Omelette (page 74)
- Quick-Mix Pancakes (page 78)

Lunches are a wonderful opportunity to brown bag a healthy meal as an alternative to fast food or ordering in. You can certainly get a "two-for-one" if you make extra at dinner the night before and lunch on healthy leftovers the next day, or save kitchen clean-up time by making tomorrow's lunch while making dinner. Some particularly convenient make-it-quick lunches are:

- Chicken Quesadillas (page 86)
- Roasted Red Pepper and Tortellini Salad (page 87)
- Turkey Tortilla Roll (page 89)
- Mango-Chicken Salad Sandwiches (page 90)

- Dilled Tortilla Roll (page 91)
- Vegetable Tortilla Pizza (page 92)
- English Muffin Pizza (page 92)
- Spinach and Mushroom Pita Pizza (page 93)
- Guiltless Nachos (page 93)
- Chicken Confetti Salad (page 94)
- Market Club Sandwich (page 95)
- Pasta and Chickpea Soup (page 100)
- Smoked Turkey and White Bean Soup (page 100)
- Chili in a Hurry (page 102)

If preparing more dinners is your goal, you certainly don't need to plan and shop for seven full menus each week. Factor in meals out and the meals you might have in the freezer, or those quick meals when evening schedules don't allow a leisurely sit-down dinner with the family or friends. If you've been doing very little home cooking and have a realistic goal of making one or two dinners a week, perhaps you can cook on the weekend when you have the time. Some particularly make-it-snappy dinners are:

- Bowtie Pasta With Wild Mushroom Sauce (page 108)
- Risotto With Spring Vegetables (page 109)
- Breast of Chicken Nicoise (page 113)
- Chicken Curry Over Rice (page 116)
- Chicken Paella (page 117)
- Turkey Carbonara (page 121)
- Chicken Au Poivre (page 123)
- Veal Picatta (page 125)
- Pasta Shrimp Pomodoro (page 143)
- Herb-Crusted Orange Roughy (page 147)
- Roasted Cod With Vegetables (page 149)
- Shrimp Salad St. Lucia (page 151)
- Pan-Roasted Crab Cakes (page 153)
- Poached Salmon (page 155)
- Herbed Shrimp Pasta Primavera (page 157)

make it
healthy;
make it
quick

My Quickest Meals

These are my "go to" meals when time is simply not there to do anything beyond assemble or heat and go!

1. **Cheese Quesadillas:** Fat-free, whole-wheat tortilla sprinkled with 2 oz. shredded part-skim-milk cheddar cheese and drizzled with salsa—folded and browned in nonstick skillet till cheese melts. Serve with fresh mango or apple slices.

2. **Baked Spaghetti:** Cooked whole-wheat angel hair pasta in a sheet pan—topped with one jar of Classico Tomato Basil Sauce and sprinkled with 1 lb. of shredded part-skim-milk mozzarella cheese and baked for 8–10 minutes at 375 degrees. One three- by five-inch slice (index card size) is approximately one serving. Serve with "Salad in a Bag" served with low-fat vinaigrette.

3. **Vegetable Tortilla Pizza (page 92):** Large whole-wheat flour tortilla brushed with Classico's Tomato Basil Sauce and topped with chopped veggies of choice and sprinkled with grated part-skim-milk mozzarella cheese. Bake until lightly browned and crisp (about 5 minutes) at 450 degrees. Serve with baby carrots to munch on.

4. **Grilled Chicken Sandwich:** Grilled, marinated chicken breast (from your freezer!) on whole-grain bun with lettuce, tomato, salsa or Dijon mustard. Serve with fresh or frozen grapes.

5. **Smoked Turkey and White Bean Soup (page 100):** Smoked turkey breast (pre-cooked) made into soup with chicken stock and cannelini beans. Serve with raw vegetable platter and herbed yogurt dip.

6. **Quick Taco Salad:** Canned black beans (rinsed), spiced with creole seasoning and sprinkled with shredded part-skim-milk cheddar cheese. Heat and serve over mixed greens. Top with crumbled baked Tostitos chips with salsa. Serve with sliced naval oranges.

7. **Even Quicker Greek Salad:** Mixed greens (from a bag!) topped with crumbled feta cheese, shredded Boar's Head turkey or ham and drizzled with low-fat vinaigrette. Serve with toasted, petite, whole-wheat pita bread and a piece of fruit.

8. **Cheese-Baked Potatoes:** Microwave potatoes for 4 minutes each. Cut open and top with cooked broccoli florets and 1/2 cup preshredded, part-skim-milk cheese. Microwave again until cheese melts. Top with nonfat sour cream or salsa. Serve with salad and low-fat vinaigrette.

9. **Turkey Tortilla Roll:** Spread a whole-wheat, flour tortilla with Dijon mustard. Top with sliced Boar's Head turkey and shredded lettuce, tomatoes and red pepper strips. Roll up burrito style.

Trimming Time by Freezing Food

One way to streamline your food preparation is to look for the recipes that can be doubled or tripled, then frozen for later use. Nothing can calm frenzied nerves after a busy day—overflowing into a busy night—like a meal that can be pulled out of the freezer and heated up in a jiffy!

If you're marinating and grilling two chicken breasts, why not do a dozen? Then you can freeze them individually in small plastic zip-top bags. Later they can be popped into the microwave for quick chicken sandwiches or salads. When making French toast, I quadruple the recipe and use an entire loaf of bread—freezing the grilled toasts into individual bags. On early mornings, they can be popped out of the freezer and into the toaster for a very quick—but delicious—breakfast. The same goes for any number of dishes—from lasagna to meatloaf.

I also use this theory when I'm picking up takeout. Rather than getting two healthy Chinese meals to bring home, I bring home four. I freeze the two extras in small bags for quick meals. Combined with my own just-made brown rice, it makes a terrific mealtime treat weeks later.

So keep your eyes and mind open for doubling up on recipes, saving you time and effort later. Highlight those recipes to remind you even before you go to the store. Choose wisely which foods to freeze—some just don't freeze well. The higher the fat content of a food, the shorter its storage potential. And foods that are high in water content will turn to mush—like tomatoes, lettuce and other salad vegetables. Milk and yogurt sauces curdle when frozen.

How to Make Freezing a Breeze

In an era that has perfected living in space, you'd think that freezing muffins would be easy. But all too often food comes out of the freezer trapped in a block of ice. And when it thaws, it's soggy and tastes like the chili you defrosted last week.

Freezing preserves freshness, but it doesn't work miracles! The fresher the food when you freeze it, the better it will taste when you defrost, heat and eat it.

Use these tips:

- Cool food quickly before you freeze it. Don't let your flavor-packed, texture-filled food sit around and lose its quality. Put it in the freezing container, seal it, then cool it in very cold water before freezing.

- Pack it small. I use quart-size, heavy-duty, sealable plastic freezer bags, which can be cleaned and used again and again. Then I pack in individual portion sizes so that I can prepare for one, two or four. A whole pan of lasagna is only helpful if I'm preparing for a crowd.

- Pack it flat. Fill bags with food, press out the excess air, seal and then freeze so they are flat. The less air that's trapped in the package, the better. If you do a lot of freezing, think about investing in a home vacuum-packaging system—they're expensive but worth it.

- The faster the food freezes, the better its quality will be preserved. Freeze portions in smaller containers with lots of cold-air space circulating around them. Stack containers after they have frozen. I place the bags in boxes according to proteins, grains and vegetables. Just a simple shoebox will do!

- Foods keep best if your freezer is set at

0 degrees Fahrenheit or below. It won't spoil above that, but the quality and nutrient content will suffer greatly. Generally, if your freezer can't keep frozen yogurt brick hard, it's not cold enough. Use a hardware store refrigerator-freezer thermometer to check the temperature occasionally. Warmer than desired freezers may mean overcrowding, problems with the seal or with the freezer itself.

Freezing Points

Proper wrapping, sealing and labeling will ensure that your food retains its quality and texture after freezing, and the flavor won't wane before you use it. To do it right:

- Store foods in materials designed and designated for freezer storage, such as sturdy plastic containers, sealed plastic bags and heavy-duty plastic wrap. (Regular plastic wrap is too thin to protect foods in the freezer.)

- Make sure the seal on the wrap or container is airtight (to stave off freezer burn) and moisture proof (to stop ice crystals from forming).

- If you plan to freeze meat for more than two weeks, overwrap the store packaging with freezer wrap or seal the whole package inside a freezer bag (like zip-top freezer bags). Same for bread—and be sure to completely cool home-baked breads before packaging to prevent ice crystals from turning your creation into a soggy ball. Freeze fruit in a plastic container or bag after you have sliced and seeded it.

- Label foods before you freeze them and record a "good until" expiration date on the label rather than the date when you froze the food. Although certain foods might make the quality cut after a year or more, generally three to six months is about what to expect. Again, it's not dangerous to eat the frozen food if it's been in the big chill longer, but the flavors and textures will seriously deteriorate.

make it healthy; make it quick

What NOT to Freeze

- *Raw celery*
- *Corn on the cob*
- *Cream cheese*
- *Eggs in the shell*
- *Garlic*
- *Hard-boiled eggs*
- *Luncheon meats*
- *Mayo-based salads*
- *Potatoes*
- *Salad dressings*
- *Salad greens*
- *Sour cream*
- *Raw tomatoes*
- *Yogurt*

make it healthy; make it quick

What About Freezer Burn?

Freezer burn is a discolored, dried-out area on the surface of frozen food caused by direct exposure to desert-dry freezer air. It's fine to eat food with freezer burn— just cut off the affected portion because it will taste awful.

Invest in ice-cube trays—not for water, but for the perfect portioning they provide. Freeze small quantities of food you cook with—chicken or beef stock, tomato paste, leftover wine, single servings of marinara sauce or pesto, leftover egg whites. Use the standard segment kind for freezing, then transfer the "cubes" to easy-to-store freezer bags. You'll be able to use a cube as needed, rather than have to open or defrost a whole container.

It's also critical to defrost carefully. Don't ever leave food out at room temperature for more than three hours to thaw. Thaw overnight in the refrigerator or microwave on defrost (30 percent power) for six to eight minutes per pound of food.

Combine a frozen meal item with a fresh food—like a thawed grilled chicken breast with a fresh salad, or a thawed pasta dish topped with hot seared seafood. This will give you a great balance of aroma, nutrients and texture.

After a month of cooking for your immediate meal, plus making extra to store in the freezer, it won't be necessary to cook but two to three times a week—because there is always something special waiting for you in the freezer!

Stocking Up Trims Time

As flavorful, simple and inexpensive as making your own stocks, sauces—even salads—can be, there are healthy, time-saving ingredients in your grocery store that can put convenience at your hand's reach:

CHICKEN STOCKS: Try Swanson Natural Goodness low-sodium, fat-free chicken broth— it's really "chickeny" without any aftertaste.

CANNED BEANS: Try Goya or Eden Organic. The adzuki beans and the soybeans, as well as all the usual black and white ones, are tasty and quick. Just rinse and drain in colander and proceed as if they were just cooked.

FROZEN, COOKED SHRIMP: Having a bag of these already peeled and deveined in the freezer is as handy as having a can of tuna in the pantry.

FRUIT JUICES: 100 percent pure juices (look for "no sugar added") are on your grocer's shelves, close to the dairy cases. They make wonderful marinades, bringing out the flavor of foods such as poultry and seafood. You can also buy frozen juice concentrates and use them as natural sweeteners to replace refined sugar.

MARINADE: A quick and easy marinade that is great for chicken, pork, fish and seafood is Lea and Perrins Worcestershire for Chicken. Just fifteen minutes will add a great boost of flavor to your meats.

PACKAGED, WASHED AND PREPPED SALAD PACKS AND FRESH VEGETABLES: Now that producers are bagging shredded carrots, broccoli florets, cauliflower and prewashed lettuces, there's no time excuse for not eating your veggies and salads. Yes, they cost more than whole heads of lettuce and bags of whole carrots—but you'll eat a lot more of them this way! The salads are ready to eat, and the vegetables work wonders for quick stir-fry and fresh vegetable platters.

PASTA SAUCE: Try Classico or Barillo. Of all the jarred sauces, these nongoopy, not-too-sweet, just-the-right-garlic formulas are best. They are made from naturally fresh ingredients with less than 2 grams of fat per serving.

PRESHREDDED, 2 PERCENT MILK CHEDDAR OR MOZZARELLA CHEESE

CHEESES: The convenience of grated hard cheeses (like Parmesan) isn't worth the compromise in flavor, but buying bags of preshredded, semi-soft cheeses makes sense. Store brands work just as well as Kraft or Sargento—just look for part-skim milk or 2 percent fat cheese.

ROASTED RED PEPPERS OR CANNED WHOLE CHILIES: The jarred version tastes like the homemade version of fresh peppers you blacken under the broiler, steam, peel, core, seed and slice—if you had time. The peppers are bottled with water in 7 1/2-ounce or larger jars, and can usually be found alongside other Italian items in supermarkets.

Convenience products such as these provide the opportunity for minimal kitchen work. Most people really don't hate to cook; what they hate is the stress and spending more time in the kitchen—particularly cleaning up more mess.

Healthy home cooking is still possible—even if you are living life in the express lane! Keeping a well-stocked pantry, planning a week's worth of healthy menus and knowing some shortcuts can simplify weekday meal preparation enough to make it, if not a joy, at least less of a hassle. Save even more time by letting the supermarket salad bars supply you with diced or cubed fresh fruits and veggies—you can buy exactly the amount you need. I also get peeled, freshly cooked shrimp from the seafood counter and fresh grilled chicken breasts from the deli. Healthy home cooking is cheaper and more nutritious, and you can control the calories and fat a lot better.

The point of healthy cooking is a simple one—good living. It's not just about solving weight or disease issues alone—it's about releasing energy for life. And that is the foundation upon which all of these recipes and meal ideas are built.

Rather than this being a health book that tells you what not to eat, this healthy cookbook focuses on what to eat—and why. Next you'll find an Eat Right Prescription and How-To Guide for a life filled with good health and good food.

make it healthy; make it quick

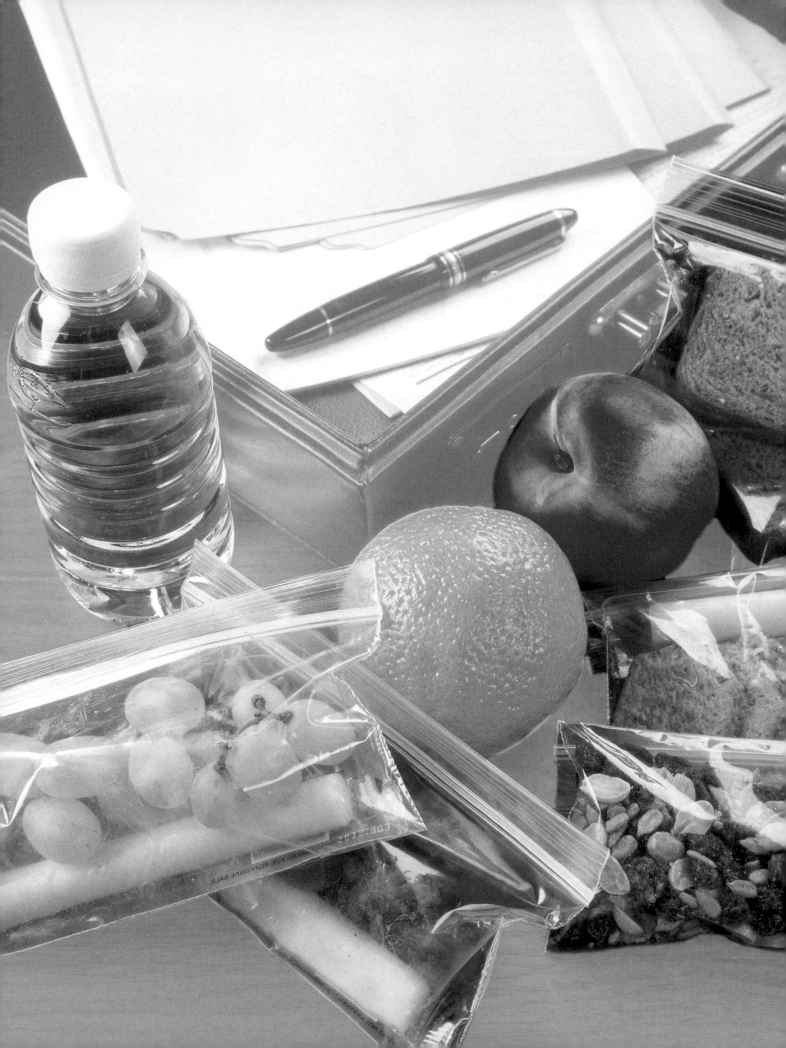

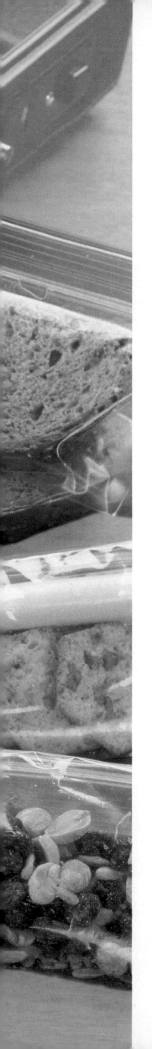

good living: the foundation

Do you ever feel as if there's a conspiracy to keep you confused about good eating for good health? If so, you're not alone! Daily newspapers, popular magazines, radio and TV talk shows all promote a wide range of opinions and theories. It seems almost impossible to separate fact from fiction.

How can I have more energy? How do I lose weight and keep it off? How do I keep my cholesterol and blood pressure in check? How can I take charge of the stresses of life—or my hormones? These are the questions many of us ask about nutritious eating.

But today's fad diet designers cannot answer these questions. Instead, we need to consider how our bodies were designed to be fed and fueled.

Our problem is not just that we're eating unhealthy food or even that we're eating too much. It's that most of us push our bodies through the day, living on fumes rather than fuel. When we finally eat, it's too much too late.

We are caught in a trap of too much to do and too little time in which to do it—life in this twenty-first century has become complex and super-stressful. It requires a continuous supply of nutritious food to meet those never-ceasing demands. We need the right foods at the right time and in the right balance just to survive—let alone thrive—in the midst of stress.

The stresses of living life in the fast lane make your body respond as if your life were threatened. It reads your stress as a danger signal—and it sets off automatic chemical reactions within your body to prepare you to flee or fight this present danger.

These chemical reactions result in many of the present-day maladies of life: fatigue, obesity, diabetes, ulcers and gastrointestinal distress, hypertension, high levels of cholesterol and triglycerides, raging hormones, migraines—even depression. And, this stressful lifestyle has slowed our metabolic rates to a snail's pace, resulting in fats being stored rather than burned for energy.

Couple these reactions with the reality that most of us are underfueled and underfed, that

Pictured: Power snacks (pg. 17)

good living: the foundation

we push our bodies through the day without food much like pushing a car uphill without gasoline, and it's not hard to understand why we are overcome with the stresses of life—and have no energy for healthy cooking. It's understandable why our metabolisms stay stuck in low gear, storing away every meal as if it were our last. We are busy and tired, but more than likely too busy or too tired to do anything about it.

Join with me as we navigate through the troubled waters of our busy lives and learn how to answer the "what abouts…" that get us off the course of wellness and often leave us shipwrecked. Unlike the diets you may have followed in the past, I put emphasis on eating—what to eat (rather than what to avoid), when to eat and why you should be eating it. You can count the calories and nutrients taken in, but what really matters is which calories are burned and which nutrients are used. To get our bodies working with us and for us, we need to eat early, eat often, eat balanced and bright, and eat lean. In the following pages, I explain each of these four key concepts in detail.

1. Eat Early

Your mother was right—you do need breakfast! Breakfast calories are like a smart investment: The return is greater than the initial deposit.

We don't save calories by skipping breakfast. On the contrary, because breakfast starts up our metabolisms for the new day, it helps ensure that the rest of the day's calories are burned more efficiently—as energy—rather than stored as fat. Breakfast also increases our ability to concentrate and keeps our appetites under control.

Our bodies respond differently to small meals than big meals. After a big meal, the body puts out an excess of insulin, which is a fat storage hormone. Extra insulin prevents fat cells from releasing fatty acid into the bloodstream where it can be picked up by other tissues and burned for energy. In other words, excess insulin released at large meals causes fat to be stored in the body rather than used for energy.

Eating smaller meals more often is a lot like throwing logs on our slow-burning metabolic fires, helping them burn better and brighter. It all starts with breakfast. We must "break the fast" with breakfast to rev up the body. If you miss this vital meal, you'll be running with no fuel for sixteen to eighteen hours, the time since your last meal—probably dinner the night before. You drag through the day tired, irritable, unmotivated and unable to concentrate. Who wants to have a day like that?

Remember that breakfast does not have to be a time-robber—it is actually a time-giver. Because a smart breakfast stabilizes your blood chemistries, you will have more energy and alertness, and you will even be able to think more clearly.

Breakfast makes you more productive and effective, helping you do what you do quickly, with fewer mistakes. How's that for a wise time investment?

You may not feel hungry in the morning. If that's the case, you simply need to wake up your natural appetite with a balanced breakfast. Breakfast will neutralize the body's blood sugars and stomach acids and get you out of that early morning slowed-down state.

Do you complain that eating breakfast makes you feel hungry throughout the day? It should. Not only does starving in the morning slow your metabolism, but the result is the use of your own tissue for energy. This deprivation releases waste products into your system that temporarily depress your appetite and give you a feeling of fullness. You can continue to starve without feeling hungry for hours. Sadly, this backfires later in the day.

The reason you get hungry so soon after you have eaten breakfast is that you have taken yourself out of the starved mode and lifted up your blood sugars. What goes up will come down. Even with a correctly balanced breakfast your blood sugar will crest and fall within three hours or so. (That's the time to have a power snack!)

If you have early morning appointments or an on-the-go family with little time for breakfast, eat breakfast on the run if you must. It can be a meal as simple as toast with melted cheese, fruited yogurt with a muffin, or whole-grain cereal and fruit with skim milk. Even a turkey sandwich or slice of pizza will do. The key is to eat and eat soon—within a half-hour after getting up from your night's sleep.

Plan a breakfast plate that is balanced. A balanced breakfast supplies adequate carbohydrates and protein—you can't live well on the fumes from a piece of toast or a cup of coffee.

Serve three different foods at breakfast: a quick energy-starting simple carbohydrate (fruit or juice), a long-lasting complex carbohydrate (grains, cereal, bread or muffins) and a power-building protein (dairy, eggs or meats).

POWER SNACK CHOICES

Baked Tostitos or Guiltless Gourmet tortilla chips with $\frac{1}{3}$ cup fat-free bean dip and salsa

$\frac{1}{2}$ sandwich on whole-grain kaiser roll or whole-wheat bread, made with: turkey and mozzarella (with light mayo and touch of mustard) or ham and fat-free cheese (with light mayo and touch of mustard)

Whole-grain cereal with skim milk

Date Cheese Spread (pg. 67) and whole-grain crackers

Charlie's Lunch Kit or small pop-top can of tuna with whole-grain crackers

Harvest Crisps crackers or Raisin Squares cereal with Laughing Cow Light cheese wedge or low-fat string cheese

Health Valley graham crackers or whole-wheat bread with 2 Tbsp. natural peanut butter

Crispbread crackers with sliced turkey and Dijon mustard

Light popcorn with 2 Tbsp. fresh grated Parmesan cheese

Stonyfield Farm yogurt or plain, nonfat yogurt mixed with all-fruit spread

12 grapes or 10 fresh strawberries with low-fat string cheese or Armenian cheese

Gazpacho in cups with low-fat string cheese

Fruit shake (skim milk blended with frozen fruit and vanilla)

Low-fat cheese tortellini salad in vinaigrette with carrots and celery

Dill tortilla rolls: whole-wheat tortilla with fat-free cream cheese, lemon juice, fresh dill and creole seasoning

Trail mix (1 cup unsalted, dry-roasted peanuts or soy nuts; 1 cup unsalted, dry-roasted, shelled sunflower or pumpkin seeds; and 2 cups raisins—make in abundance and bag into $\frac{1}{4}$ or $\frac{1}{2}$ cup portions)

Homemade low-fat bran muffin (pg. 66) and skim milk

good living: the foundation

Again, don't be concerned if the meals are not made up of traditional choices. There is nothing wrong with pizza for breakfast or cereal for dinner! Just remember, the best breakfast foods are the ones that you will eat.

Try some of the "grab and go" breakfasts beginning on page 64. They are designed to stoke up your metabolism and start your day with boundless energy to meet the demands placed upon you. They make breakfast time-efficient and delicious!

2. Eat Often

Once you start with breakfast, eating mini-meals often throughout the day, about every two-and-a-half to three hours, will keep your metabolism and energy burning high and your appetite in better control. This power snacking also stabilizes insulin to low levels in the bloodstream—meaning less fat will be stored and more energy and more fat will be burned. That's good news!

Once you start power snacking, your body will reward you with higher energy and metabolism levels.

Many of us have grown up with a three-square-meals mentality, thinking snacks are harmful. Yet the truth about snacking is this: Wisely chosen snacks are a necessary part of a healthy diet, not a special treat or an afterthought.

One of the biggest health mistakes you can make is to starve throughout the day, saving up calories for the evening. This throws off your metabolism and sets you up for binge-like eating.

Above all else, remember your body was created to survive. It reads long hours without food as starvation and will slow your metabolic rate to preserve your valuable muscle mass. Then it plays a trick on itself and turns first to the muscle mass for energy and last to your fat stores!

Several small meals deposit less fat than one or two large meals, even if you eat the same amount of the same foods. And smaller, more frequent meals will create more energy, leaner bodies and better blood chemistries. Power snacking prevents plummeting blood sugars that leave you grouchy and craving sweets.

I plan my day to include three meals and three to four snacks (one midmorning; one or two midafternoon, depending on the lateness of the dinner hour; and one bedtime snack). By planning to eat the right foods at the right times, you gain freedom from the constant battle that can rage between your appetite and your eating, lack of eating or compulsive overeating. Wise snacking through the day will keep an out-of-control appetite at bay!

Stock your kitchen with healthful and wise snack combos. Keep your snacks ready by placing one portion in a zip-top bag in your refrigerator or pantry. Tuck them into your briefcase or purse to take with you when you go to work.

Because healthy snacking is such a necessary part of a healthy diet, don't waste it on the typical snack foods that are low in essential nutrients yet loaded with salt, sugar, fat and calories. If only soda, chips, cookies and candy are available, that's what you will reach for. Wise

POWER PROTEINS

Each portion equals 1 ounce of protein (7 grams)

- Nonfat milk or nonfat plain yogurt . . . .4 oz.

- Low-fat cheeses . . . . .1 oz.
  (or ¼ cup grated)

- 1 percent low-fat or nonfat cottage cheese or part-skim or fat-free ricotta . . . . . .¼ cup

- Eggs (particularly use egg whites) 1

- Fish . . . . .1 oz.
  (or ¼ cup flaked fish)

- Seafood (crab, lobster) . . . . .¼ cup

- Seafood (clams, shrimp, oysters or scallops) 5

- Turkey, cornish hens . . . . .1 oz.
  (or ¼ cup chopped)

- Chicken . . . . .1 oz.
  (or ¼ cup chopped)

- Beef, pork, lamb, veal (lean, trimmed) . .1 oz.

- Legumes . . . . .¼ cup
  (Black beans, garbanzo beans, Great Northern beans, kidney beans, lentils, navy beans, peanuts, red beans, split peas, soybeans and soy products such as tofu and soy milk)

  Although a plant food, legumes contain valuable protein if eaten with a grain (corn, wheat, rice, oats) or a seed (pumpkin, sunflower, sesame).

- Natural peanut butter . . . . .2 Tbsp.

Solomon seemed to know this, writing with inspiration: "He who is full loathes honey, but to the hungry even what is bitter tastes sweet" (Prov. 27:7). No need to set these foods up as "forbidden fruit"—just focus on foods that bless your body.

Watch out for many of the fat-free foods that are becoming such a booming business. Many companies pander to the American sweet tooth and load them with sugar.

It is more nutritious to eat fresh fruit than fat-free (but probably sugar-laden) cupcakes. We need to learn to make good food choices. Manufactured foods, such as fat-free baked goods, just cultivate our taste for sweets. It makes no sense to trade a diet moderate in fat for one higher in sugar.

3. Eat Balanced and Bright

Balance is more than a wide variety of foods displayed on a pretty plate; it's giving our bodies the right foods at the right times. This means a balance of carbohydrates and proteins at every meal and snack.

These nutrients have two different yet equally vital functions. Carbohydrates are 100 percent pure energy—they are your body's fuel, designed to burn fast, clean and pure. Proteins, however, are your body's building blocks. They are designed to build lean body tissues, strengthen immunities, balance fluids and boost the metabolism.

The healthy goal is to choose carbohydrates in the most whole form possible and thus benefit from both their nutrients and fiber. This means eating whole grains when you can, such as brown rice, oats and 100 percent whole-grain

good living: the foundation

ENERGY-GIVING CARBOHYDRATES

Simple Carbohydrates
(Fruits and Nonstarchy Vegetables)

All fruits and fruit juices

Apples, apricots, bananas, berries, cherries, dates, grapefruit, grapes, kiwis, lemons, limes, melons, nectarines, oranges, peaches, pears, pineapples, plums, raisins

(Generally one serving of simple carbohydrate is obtained from ½ cup fruit, ½ cup fruit juice or ⅛ cup dried fruit. This gives 10 grams of simple carbohydrate.)

Nonstarchy vegetables

Asparagus, beets, broccoli, Brussels sprouts, cabbage, carrots, cauliflower, celery, green beans, green leafy vegetables, kale, mushrooms, okra, onions, snow peas, sugar snap peas, summer squash, tomatoes, zucchini

(Generally one serving of simple carbohydrate is obtained from ½ cup cooked vegetables or 1 cup raw vegetables or juice. This gives 10 grams of simple carbohydrate.)

Complex Carbohydrates
(Grains and Starchy Vegetables)

Grains

The following amounts provide one serving of complex carbohydrate, giving 15 grams:

Barley, bulgur, couscous, grits, kasha, millet or polenta, cooked . . . . .½ cup

Bread . . . . .1 slice

Cereals . . . . .1 oz.
(¼ cup of a concentrated cereal such as Grape-Nuts or granola, ½ to ¾ cup flaked cereals and 1 cup puffed cereals)

Crackers or mini-rice cakes 5

Crispbread or rice cakes 2

Oats, uncooked . . . . .⅓ cup

Pasta or rice, cooked . . . . .½ cup

Fat-free tortillas (flour or corn) 1

Wheat germ . . . . .¼ cup

Starchy vegetables

Black-eyed peas, corn, green peas, lima beans, parsnips, potatoes (white and sweet), rutabagas, turnips and winter squash

(Generally one serving of complex carbohydrate is obtained from ½ cup cooked starchy vegetables, giving 15 grams.)

good living: the foundation

breads, crackers, cereals and pastas. Eat fruits and vegetables well-washed with their skins on, and choose the fruit rather than the fruit juice.

In addition, choose power-building proteins in the lowest-fat form that you can, and prepare them with the lowest-fat cooking methods possible. As much as you need carbohydrates to burn and proteins to build, it's fat that makes you fat! Yet it isn't worth sacrificing your protein intake to cut back on fat. Protein is too vital to skip. Just shift to proteins that are lean or, in the case of dairy products, that are made from skim milk.

In this section I have included charts for power proteins and energy-giving carbohydrates. Be sure to include foods from these sources with every meal and snack. Generally a meal should give 2–3 ounces of protein and at least one serving of a complex and simple carbohydrate. A snack should provide 1–2 ounces of protein and one serving of carbohydrate.

Healthy living eating is based on this essential balance. In the recipes in this book, you'll see a breakdown of complex carbohydrates and simple carbohydrates for each meal. You'll also see a strong emphasis on variety—the time-tested answer to the "How do I keep healthy?" question.

No one food is perfect; no one food contains all the nutrients we need. But be sure to provide whole-grain, low-fat meals that are full of a variety of brightly colored fruits and vegetables. The bright coloring is a sign of the nutritional content of a vegetable or fruit. Generally the more vivid the coloring, the more essential nutrients it holds. That deep orange or red coloring in carrots, sweet potatoes, cantaloupes, apricots, peaches and strawberries signals their vitamin A content. Dark green, leafy vegetables such as greens, spinach, romaine lettuce, Brussels sprouts and broccoli are loaded with vitamin A as well as folic acid. Vitamin C is found in more than just citrus; it is also power-packed into strawberries, cantaloupes, tomatoes, green peppers and broccoli. You may not be able to tell a book by its cover, but you can tell the power of a fruit or veggie by its color!

Your health doesn't depend on a single food or a single meal. Healthy variety occurs when you make good food choices over a period of time. Because there is no one food you must have to survive, substitution is your best strategy. Mixing and matching foods for healthy variety over a period of one to two days is the name of the game.

4. Eat Lean

The story about fat has become a confusing one—from being the nutritional bad guy of the nineties to being applauded as the way to lose weight by fad-diet designers—it's hard to know the correct move to make when it comes to cutting the fat from our diets.

The truth about fat is this: The most up-to-date research continues to point to excess fat as paving the road to obesity and disease. The excess fat calories we consume are converted and stored as fat more readily than those from other sources. Fat is a more concentrated source of calories (all fats contain twice as many calories as equal amounts of carbohydrates or proteins, about 9 calories per gram or 120 calories per tablespoon). In healthy weight loss, trimming the fat is as important as trimming calories.

Of course, fatness or thinness is not the only factor involved in food choices. Even if you have been blessed with a metabolism that burns brightly, allowing you to maintain your weight easily, excess fat intake can cause health problems. You may not see the problems on the scale or your waistline, but you'll want to consider these vital facts about fat and your health. Excess fat intake, particularly saturated fat, increases your cholesterol and blood pressure levels and your risk of heart disease and stroke, regardless of your weight. It has been indicated in cancer and gallbladder disease, in addition to increasing the susceptibility to diabetes to those genetically inclined.

An important reality—preventing the diseases of tomorrow is wonderful, but the reason to change is for today! Eating a balanced diet low in fat, particularly saturated fats, yet high in whole grains, fruits and vegetables, gives us higher levels of energy and alertness, better stress management and even improved memory and sleep. These are the reasons I prescribe a low-fat eating plan for even my thinnest clients.

The facts point to a less-is-more lifestyle choice: Less fat in our diet means more wellness and protection from disease and weight struggles. Of course, entering this low-fat lifestyle can be tricky when it is estimated that today's American takes in approximately 40 percent of his daily calories from fat. Chances are good that you may be eating more than you realize. A typical adult eats the fat equivalent of one stick of butter a day!

The first line of defense in any battle is to identify your enemies. In the war against excess fat, the enemy's hideouts are meats, poultry, whole-fat dairy products and nuts, along with butter and oil toppings. Fruits, vegetables and grains have little or no fat, as long as they aren't fattened up with butters and sauces.

I was raised on fried chicken, mashed potatoes and gravy, and green beans cooked in bacon grease. Maybe you were, too. Embracing a lifestyle of better eating and better living meant a lot more to me than cutting candy bars—it meant finding ways to enjoy flavorful foods without grease. I wasn't about to accept a life filled with dry, tasteless foods that resemble cardboard—so I had to establish new ways of shopping, cooking and dining out. Techniques or ingredients are different from traditional cooking in cooking great-tasting, lower-fat meals. As an example, fat plays an important role in cooking and baking, so it is difficult simply to omit it. It acts as a flavor enhancer and gives food a distinctive and desirable texture.

With that said, I don't banish all butter, oil and other types of fat from my recipes. Instead I use small amounts of the highest possible quality. The greatest proportion of any fat I use is extra-virgin olive oil, and fats are added at just the right moment to maximize the flavor.

I employ several techniques to enhance flavor and texture, without excess fat:

- Using herbs, spices and flavorful vegetables in a variety of combinations

- "Sautéing" vegetables in a small amount of broth to further reduce the need for oil; caramelizing them to draw out their natural sweetness and flavoring

- Using nonstick cookware and nonstick cooking spray to reduce the need for added fats

- Choosing alternative protein sources such as legumes in recipes—often using meat as an accent flavor rather than the star attraction

You'll find many more of these tips, tricks and low-fat substitutions in the next chapter, "Good Cooking."

HOW MUCH IS ENOUGH?

Experts recommend limiting fat intake to between 25 and 30 percent of total calorie limit. Moderately active women need approximately 2,000 calories daily for maintaining weight; moderately active men need 2,500 calories. For weight loss goals, a good daily limit for women is 1,200 calories; for men, 1,500 calories. To determine the 25 percent fat allowance, use this formula:

25 percent x 1,200 calories = 300 calories
300 calories ÷ 9 calories per gram of fat =
33 grams maximum fat suggested each day.

Daily Calories	Grams of Fat per Day
1,200 calories	33 grams
1,500 calories	42 grams
1,800 calories	50 grams
2,000 calories	56 grams
2,500 calories	69 grams

What About Salt?

Although salt is certainly not the number one nutritional evil, it is nonetheless a concern. The main problem is how much we use of it—way, way too much! Actually, the average American consumes more than eight times his or her daily requirement—about fifteen pounds per year. This is the sodium equivalent of two to four teaspoons of salt a day.

Hypertension, fluid retention and kidney dysfunction are just a few of the health problems those little white granules contribute to—good reasons to pass on the salt!

In America today, approximately sixty million people have abnormally high blood pressure. This means that one person out of five is predisposed to the condition. However, it's not possible to identify who is at risk, so it's wise to practice prevention and cut back on excess salt—even before a doctor tells you that you must. An ounce of prevention can be worth a pound of cure.

good living: the foundation

good living: the foundation

Watch Out for High-Sodium Foods

- *Any food pickled or brine-cured, including sauerkraut, pickles and olives*

- *Any food salt-cured or smoked, including most ham, bacon and sausage*

- *Any cold cuts, including bologna, hot dogs, pastrami and salami*

- *Convenience foods, such as canned vegetables, soups and frozen meals*

Salt is made up of 60 percent sodium and 40 percent chloride. In the human body, excess sodium becomes a troublemaker, creating a temporary buildup of fluids, making it harder for the heart to pump blood through the system and causing a rise in the blood pressure (hypertension). Other factors besides salt intake, such as heredity and obesity, can also contribute to hypertension. Unlike heredity, however, salt consumption is a factor within our control. Unfortunately, for the majority of Americans it is out of control.

Shaking the salt habit can be difficult because of our taste buds. They were designed to pick up the taste of salt in foods, but our high-salt diets have overdeveloped that desire. We weren't born loving salt—but by being given salted foods, we began to prefer them. The good news is that this conditioned taste is reversible: As you use less salt, your tastes will change so that you will enjoy foods more without so much salt. It takes only six weeks or so to see a big difference in salt desire.

Salt does play a big part in food's enjoyment; it serves as a catalyst for flavor, enhancing the taste of ingredients. The key to making the good-for-you cutback is to learn to prepare foods in ways that naturally enhance the flavor so they need less salt to taste good. You'll notice *Healthy Living* recipes use herbs and spices, which allow you to reduce the amount of salt drastically.

What About Additives and Preservatives?

Serving hot dogs and cold cuts is an easy trap to fall into—and one to be avoided! Bacon, hot dogs, sausages and the like are all high in saturated fats and sodium, and they contain nitrites, which are linked to cancer, and other chemical additives. There are far better sources for protein than these. Consider the wonderful building proteins on page 18.

I advocate "real foods" rather than highly processed packaged foods. For example, real orange juice or frozen concentrate is a far superior choice to fortified orange-flavored drink.

Think "Mother Nature" when you shop. Your grocery store is crammed full of healthful foods; you don't have to shop at a health food store to get them.

What About Cholesterol?

You need cholesterol for many body functions. It's necessary for hormone production, digestion, even efficient operation of the brain—but you don't have to eat it to have it. Your body makes plenty, often too much, all on its own. The liver produces cholesterol, and those with a genetic tendency toward heart disease may have a liver that produces too much and a body that metabolizes too little.

Dangerous levels of cholesterol come from eating too much of the kind of cholesterol that comes from animal products such as meat, chicken, eggs, milk, cheese and butter. More commonly, cholesterol levels in the blood rise from eating a diet high in saturated fats, which can convert to a bad form of cholesterol—LDL cholesterol.

When at a high level in the bloodstream, LDL cholesterol tends to deposit in the walls of the blood vessels, especially those in the heart, leading to arteriosclerosis, or "hardening of the arteries." The "good" form of cholesterol (HDL) has just the opposite effect: It protects the body by pulling the bad cholesterol, like a magnet, from the bloodstream.

What About Artificial Sweeteners?

As you become aware (and possibly alarmed) about your intake of sugar, you may be tempted to use sugar substitutes as a replacement. Be careful not to do this. There are no absolutes in the safety of chemicals—saccharin, aspartame or any new one to come along. The long-term effects of their use will not be known for years. As bad as sugar may be, and whatever the health hazards associated with its overuse, at least it's not a chemical. It has been used for centuries. The best wisdom to use is, "When in doubt, leave it out."

We don't eat desserts on a regular basis at our house, preferring to end our meals with fresh fruits, God's natural provision for our sweet tooth. I have included dessert recipes here, however, to complete certain menus and make them special for festive events.

But you won't find elaborate desserts in this book. Quick tricks with fresh fruits, frozen yogurts and fresh fruit sauces give you the opportunity for a fun and flavorful end to any meal.

TIPS FOR AVOIDING
THE CHOLESTEROL TRAP

- **Eat breakfast; follow with power snacks.**
  Eat small amounts of food, evenly distributed throughout the day. Starving through the day results in a metabolism that is more apt to store cholesterol than clear it from the body.

- **Eat high-fiber foods.**
  Include brown rice, legumes, oat bran and barley in your diet. Foods high in pectin, such as strawberries and bananas, slow the absorption of cholesterol into the bloodstream.

- **Eat more fish.**
  Fish contains wonderfully healthy EPA oils that lower total cholesterol and triglycerides while increasing the levels of good HDL cholesterol.

- **Eat onions and garlic.**
  These appear to raise HDL cholesterol levels dramatically, along with lowering the LDL cholesterol levels.

- **Eat very little fat.**
  The fat you eat should be monounsaturated oils, such as olive and canola oils. Avoid saturated animal and hydrogenated vegetable fats and the highly saturated coconut and palm oils.

- **Exercise aerobically.**
  Best results come from an hour of aerobic exercise every other day.

- **Lose body fat.**
  A lower body-fat percentage will help control cholesterol and triglyceride levels.

- **If you smoke, stop.**
  Each cigarette you smoke raises your cholesterol level.

What About Caffeine?

As hard as it is to imagine, caffeine, a relatively mild stimulant, is among the world's most widely used and addictive drugs. And like any drug, there is a downside to caffeine. Because it's a central nervous system stimulant, even small amounts of it can cause side effects such as restlessness, disturbed sleep, stomach irritation and diarrhea. It can cause irritability, anxiety and mood disturbances.

The amount required to cause these effects is 250 milligrams—about two mugs of coffee or three large glasses of tea. That adds up quickly, especially when you consider all of the other hidden sources of caffeine. Along with coffee and tea, caffeine is found in chocolate, sodas and some decongestants and aspirins.

Generally, the cola beverages have the highest levels of caffeine, but read all labels, since some of the fruit-flavored sodas contain caffeine as well. Some, such as Mountain Dew and Dr. Pepper, contain as much caffeine as coffee and tea. In the body of a 60-pound child, one of these sodas is the equivalent to the caffeine in four cups of coffee for a 175-pound man. Of course, the major problem with soda is not the caffeine; it's the artificial flavors, artificial colorings and the incredibly high concentration of sugar! Most sodas contain 10 to 12 teaspoons of sugar per can; the diet sodas simply replace the sugar with chemicals.

Getting Started

One last point to remember: It's your day-to-day eating that counts most for health and wellness—not what you eat at a ball game or on your birthday. One day, even a week, of less-than-great eating will not send your body headfirst into disease or nutrient deficiency.

What is important is getting started with the energy and excitement of a new way of eating! It's progress, not perfection, that counts. You may start with eating breakfast, perhaps for the first time since you were five years old. Or you may start packing a more interesting lunch that's healthier, too. It may be one fabulous dinner a week or elements of health sprinkled throughout your life.

Whatever you choose as your first step, the rewards of better eating come quickly: terrific energy, resistance to infection, good moods, superior concentration, alertness and even a better memory!

Get on with healthy living, and get cooking!

good living: the foundation

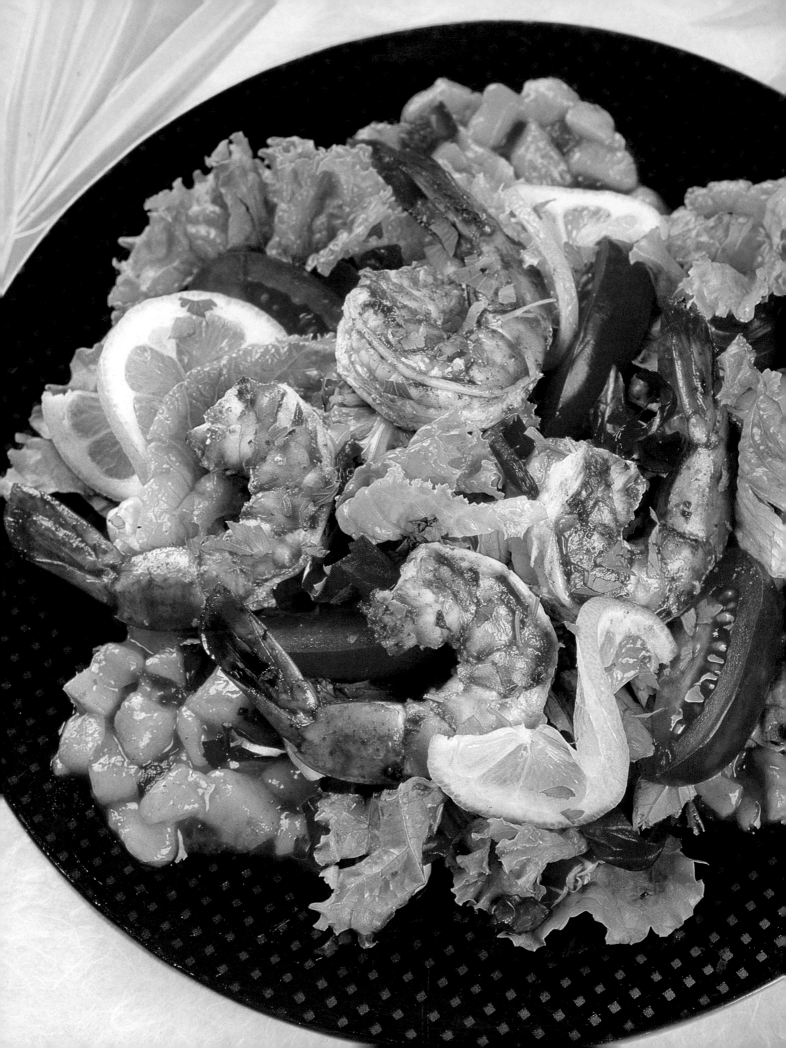

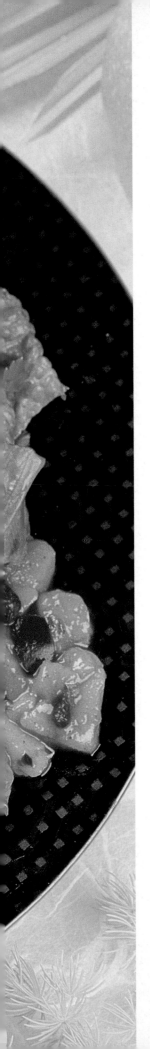

good cooking

The art of cooking doesn't start or stop at the stove. It begins with planning meals and shopping for food, and carries through to the presentation.

The recipes and meals you'll find here are designed for beauty as you serve them. Healthy living and cooking is more than just a nutritionally balanced plate; it's also a satisfying and beautiful plate. You'll find exciting new meal ideas and light versions of contemporary classics—all created with an eye for health. There are recipes for every meal and event—even mouthwatering desserts. Every dish is remarkably low in fat, particularly the saturated type. There is at-a-glance nutritional information for every recipe so you can see at once just what it contains. Whether you are on a special diet or just trying to live better, this is an indispensable guide to healthy, happy and completely satisfying eating and entertaining.

If you have even a few cooking skills, making dishes from this cookbook will be a breeze.

But please remember that these recipes are not set in stone—if you are not feeling very adventurous or industrious, you may want to simplify them even further by leaving out some herbs, spices and garnishes in some of the fancier recipes and taking a simple approach. The main ingredients and basic preparation will provide you with excellent nourishment and flavor on their own. If, on the other hand, you are feeling quite enthusiastic about cooking, you may want to follow the recipes to the letter—they are terrific!

Substitute green beans if you aren't craving asparagus; leave off a sauce if you don't have time to make it. You can also use healthy foods you have on hand to create something new and personally yours.

Pictured: Shrimp Salad St. Lucie (pg. 151)

good cooking

Recipe Makeovers

Most of the recipes in the pages ahead have been my favorites, many passed on to me by friends (often chefs) and family. Some have been developed, others "made over" with health in mind. You will discover an endless array of cooking tricks—part art, part science—to turn unhealthy, full-of-fat dishes into tasty, nutritious ones.

Basically, I use three methods to reduce the amount of fat, calories and other detrimental substances in a recipe.

● I reduce the amount of high-fat, high-salt ingredients and look for ways to enhance flavor, texture and nutritive value.

● I replace a high-fat, high-salt ingredient with a different one that is lower in fat and sodium and higher in flavor.

● I use a cooking method that reduces fat yet enhances moisture and flavor.

Following are some of the specific ingredient substitutions and cooking techniques I used in creating the recipes in this book. You may want to use them on some of your own time-tested favorites.

Tips for Low-Fat Substitutions

● Use skim milk, nonfat plain yogurt, skim-milk cheese, low-fat or nonfat cottage cheese and light cream cheese instead of the higher-fat dairy products.

● Eat more fish and white meats and fewer red meats. If you eat red meats, buy lean and trim well, before and after cooking—and cook in a way that diminishes fat, such as grilling or broiling on a rack.

● Remove skin from poultry before cooking; you will cut the fat by 50 percent!

● Use cooking sprays and nonstick skillets that enable you to brown meats without grease. Sauté ingredients in stocks and broths rather than fats and oils.

● Adapt a recipe that says to baste with butter by basting with tomato or lemon juice, Lea and Perrins Worcestershire for Chicken or stock.

● Use monounsaturated oils such as canola or olive oil for salads or cooking. You can cut the amount called for in a recipe by two-thirds without sacrificing quality. For example, a recipe calling for three tablespoons of oil may be cut to one tablespoon. Depending on the recipe, the oil may be cut out altogether if cooking spray is used. Ideally, no more than one teaspoon of oil per serving should be used.

● Substitute nonfat plain yogurt, nonfat sour cream or blended-till-smooth low-fat cottage cheese or skim-milk ricotta in recipes calling for sour cream or mayonnaise. These products also make a great topping for baked potatoes, especially sprinkled with chives or grated Parmesan.

● Purchase tuna packed in water rather than oil; solid white tastes better.

● Use avocados and olives sparingly. Although vegetables, they are concentrated sources of fat. For example, five olives contain 50 calories of fat, and half an avocado gives you 180 calories of fat.

● Use legumes (dried beans and peas) as a main dish or a meat substitute; they make a high-nutrition, low-fat meal.

● Use egg whites or egg substitute in place of whole eggs (two egg whites = one egg). Egg whites are pure protein, and egg yolks are pure fat and cholesterol.

● Skim the fat from soup stocks, meat drippings and sauces. Refrigerate and remove the hardened surface layer of fat before reheating.

● Rarely, if ever, eat organ meats such as liver, sweetbreads and brains. They are loaded with cholesterol.

● Use only natural peanut butter, and even this in small amounts. Avoid commercial peanut butter at all costs. Commercial peanut butter is not much more than shortening and sugar. Fresh-ground natural peanut butter still contains fat, but it is a good source of protein. If you have trouble switching from the commercial type, begin by mixing it half and half with natural. Gradually increase the proportion of the natural until you have abandoned the commercial.

- Use small amounts of added fats. Butter may be your best choice. If you use margarine, the soft, squeeze-type corn oil is best, then tub margarine, then stick. The firmer the margarine, the more saturated it is because of the hydrogenation process.

- Use fat-free cheeses. Though they do not melt as smoothly as fattier versions, you can overcome this by finely shredding the cheese or mixing it with a reduced-fat ver-

sion. Two great blends are three parts fat-free mozzarella blended with one part Parmesan, or three parts fat-free sharp cheddar blended with one part part-skim-milk mozzarella.

- Replace one-quarter to one-half of the ground meat or poultry in a casserole or meat sauce with cooked brown rice, couscous or cooked beans.

- Use puréed cooked vegetables, such as carrots, potatoes or peppers, to thicken soups and stews instead of creams, egg yolks or roux.

- Use small amounts of fattier foods that pack a powerful flavor punch: feta cheese, Parmesan, coconut, toasted nuts and bacon or sausage made from turkey. You can always cut the quantity called for by 50 percent.

SUPER SUBSTITUTE SAVINGS

INSTEAD OF	USE	AND SAVE
1 cup whole milk	1 cup skim milk	10 gr. fat, 90 calories
1 cup heavy cream	1 cup evaporated skim milk	87 gr. fat, 783 calories
1 cup sour cream	1 cup fat-free sour cream	48 gr. fat, 432 calories
8 ounces cream cheese	8 ounces light cream cheese	39 gr. fat, 351 calories
2 ounces oil	cooking spray	60 gr. fat, 540 calories
1 ounce oil	1 teaspoon oil	25 gr. fat, 225 calories
1 pint mayonnaise	1 pint plain nonfat yogurt	352 gr. fat, 3,168 calories
6 whole eggs	12 egg whites	36 gr. fat, 324 calories, 1,644 mg. cholesterol
1 pint sour cream	1 pint plain nonfat yogurt or nonfat sour cream	89 gr. fat, 803 calories
4 ounces cheddar cheese	4 ounces reduced-fat cheddar cheese	25 gr. fat, 225 calories
8 ounces cream cheese	8 ounces fat-free cream cheese	79 gr. fat, 711 calories
1 pound ground beef (80 percent lean)	1 pound ground turkey breast	91 gr. fat, 819 calories

good cooking

- Beat egg whites until soft peaks form before folding them into baked goods; this increases the volume and tenderness.

Light Cooking Techniques

Second only to buying the best fresh foods to take advantage of their natural flavors is selecting the cooking method that best retains the natural moisture in foods. This reduces or eliminates the need for fats, oils and rich sauces.

The Asian tradition of stir-frying and steaming respects the most delicate ingredients, and quick grilling and pan searing seal in the flavors and moisture as well as retain as much of the nutritional value of the food as possible. The simpler the preparation techniques, the better—uncomplicated grilling, easy poaching, efficient steaming, flavorful pan searing and, above all, masterfully simple and quick presentation.

Grilling and broiling

Not just for weekends, grilling is an ideal cooking method, allowing foods to pick up extra flavor and to be cooked with a minimum of added fats.

When grilled over hot coals or broiled on a rack in the oven, meat, fish and poultry lose extra fat as it drips away. Remove as much fat as possible before cooking by skinning chicken and trimming all visible fat from meat; this prevents the fat from cooking into your food. Coat the broiler or grill rack with cooking spray to prevent sticking, and place the trimmed fat from steaks on the grill separately to allow better smoking and flavoring of the meat.

Marinating first is a key for flavorful grilling. Lemon juice, wine, vinegar and plain yogurt are good main ingredients for low-fat marinades. Combine with fruit juices, herbs or spices for taste. Baste frequently to keep food moist during grilling. Remember that marinades give moisture and tenderness, not fat, to the meat.

If grilling fish, choose firm-textured fish fillets or steaks that are about one-inch thick rather than thinner ones (thinner foods dry out on the grill). If frozen, the fish should be thawed first. Basting with marinade while broiling will keep the fish moist. Particularly good for grilling are snapper, sea bass, grouper, salmon, tuna and swordfish. Oysters and clams are also excellent for roasting on the grill. To roast unshucked oysters or clams, wash shells thoroughly; place on grill rack about four inches from hot coals; roast for ten to fifteen minutes or until shells begin to open; serve in shells.

Parchment cooking

By encasing the food in parchment paper, aluminum foil, cooking bags or wax paper, evaporation is greatly reduced, and the food stays naturally moist and flavorful. Natural casings that may be used are lettuce leaves, cabbage leaves and corn husks.

Special microwave cooking bags are available at most supermarkets, usually in the foil or plastic wrap section. They're great for microwaving fish or chicken.

Poaching

To poach means to immerse a food in a simmering liquid. Poaching is generally reserved for fruits, eggs, poultry and fish, but lamb and veal can be poached with delicious results.

When poaching on top of the stove, the pan should be filled with a small amount of almost simmering liquid, with the food placed in the liquid. The pan should be covered so steam doesn't escape; the steam keeps the food moist.

For oven poaching the food is placed in a small amount of liquid, covered with foil and roasted.

Always allow food to cool in the liquid. This permits the flavor to be absorbed. When poached, foods stay tender, moist and low in fats.

Some good liquids to use in poaching are chicken stock, fruit juices, lemon juice, tomato juice and wine.

Following is a general time table for poaching foods:

- Boneless breast of chicken—fifteen minutes

- Breast of chicken (with bone)—twenty-five minutes

- Fish fillets—ten to twelve minutes (until flakes with fork)

- Fruits—eight to ten minutes

Sautéing and stir-frying

Sautéing and stir-frying are both methods of light cooking with a minimum amount of oil. Vegetables keep their flavor, have a nice texture and retain those important water-soluble vitamins. By using nonstick cookware or a regular skillet coated with cooking spray, vegetables and meats can be cooked quickly, often with no fat added.

Cooking sprays allow high-heat searing and cooking without sticking. A cooking spray will "grease" the pan while adding only a minimal amount of fat. By keeping a can of this in your kitchen, you will be able to add only as much additional oil as the flavor of a dish requires and not a drop more. You won't achieve perfect browning of the foods, but you will have fine results as long as you cook at a moderate temperature.

Nonstick pans are sold everywhere, and some are much better than others. As with every other piece of equipment you buy, high quality will pay for itself in the long run. The major quality differences will not be in the non stick coating but in the thickness and sturdiness of the pans. Be sure that your nonstick pan is as heavy as possible.

In most recipes calling for foods to be sautéed, the fat can be drastically reduced or omitted. Some foods, such as green pepper and celery, will dry out if cooked with cooking spray alone, so I always use a small amount (no more than two teaspoons) of oil when sautéing them. You may also sauté them in one-half cup chicken or vegetable stock, stirring frequently to prevent burning. This adds a nice flavor to the vegetables.

Foods such as mushrooms, onions, meat, fish and poultry release some liquids as they cook and can easily be sautéed in cooking spray or a nonstick skillet without oil. Meats can also be browned in this way without using any fat.

Slice vegetables thin for sautéing and stir-frying. Meat, fish and poultry should be cut into small, even pieces. Heat the pan, add a little oil, toss in the food and shake; toss or stir the food for even browning. Cook only until the vegetables are crisp tender.

Sautéing and stir-frying in a minimum of olive or canola oil will also allow vegetables to be flavorful with a nice texture and not lose water-soluble vitamins.

Steaming

Steaming is an ideal method of cooking vegetables since it provides good retention of vitamins as well as taste. Vegetables will be more flavorful and nutritious if they are not cooked in a big pot of boiling water until limp and mushy. Steaming provides a healthy and tasty alternative.

Place vegetables in a steaming basket (inexpensive and easily purchased at any grocery store) above a small amount of water (keep one-fourth inch below the bottom of the steamer) and cover. Bring to a boil and continue to boil on medium heat until vegetables are crisp tender. Placing a garlic clove or a sliced onion in the steaming water will help to flavor the vegetables without fat or calories.

Be careful: Steam burns! Remove the cover slowly, with the opening away from you.

Boiling

If you are boiling vegetables in a traditional fashion, use these principles: 1) cook over high heat, 2) use a small amount of stock or water and 3) cook for a short period of time.

Microwaving

Microwaving is a great way to cook vegetables to retain nutrients and flavor, but you must be sure not to overcook. The best foods for microwave cooking are those high in moisture and low in fat, such as fish, poultry, vegetables and fruits. The foods that do not microwave well are those high in fat and low in moisture, such as beef, pork and lamb.

Banish the Meal-Planning Blues

How often have you eaten out because of simply not wanting to have to plan and shop for what you were going to cook? Do you dread looking through recipe books and figuring out which ones to put together for a meal? You are not alone—the meal-time blues strike us all. Yet, often our struggle is more with meal planning than with meal preparation.

That's why I've done more in this book than just supply recipes—I have put the recipes together into meals planned for important nutrients and balance, for color, for flavor and for texture. Something hard is paired with something soft, something crisp with something creamy, something round with something angular, something white with something colorful

A meal that has simple or bland flavors can bore your palate and leave you full, but not satisfied. Too many complex or strong flavors in a meal can overwhelm the taste buds and the taster—leaving you hungry for familiar comfort foods. A well-balanced meal balances sweet, savory, salty and acidic flavors. Variety in temperature of food brings appeal as well. It adds a contrast that heightens enjoyment. For example, warm, grilled seafood on a chilled salad is a celebration!

Texture is how a food feels in your mouth—crispy, crunchy, chewy or soft. Consistency is the food's density and firmness, as well as how it holds together on the plate. It's best to have variety—too many crisp, crunchy and chewy items can exhaust the eater's jaw, while too many soft or saucy items can form one big glob on the plate. Different shapes and heights also add variety to the meal.

Color makes for an exciting plate. Just as in clothing, some colors in food don't work well together. Equally, a plate with all brown foods will be as unappealing as a plate with everything soft and creamy, but a variety of colors can give each plate a pleasing appearance. It's as though each plate becomes an artist's canvas—be creative with bright colors and textures, and let the dish look fresh and alive

Garnishing Tips

One of the truest adages about food is, "You eat with your eyes first." A simple touch of garnish can turn a dull dish into a wonderful one. Garnishes add eye appeal and beauty to almost any food.

A general rule of thumb about garnishes is that they should be edible and, when possible, an ingredient that's in the dish. For example, a simple tomato wedge will add a uniqueness and beauty to a plate just because of its color and shape. If fresh cilantro is included, mince some extra to use as a garnish or arrange a whole sprig of cilantro on the dish. It doesn't take much effort to create a garnish while you're preparing the food.

Lots of specialized garnishing tools are available, but you'll create the most beautiful food with just a knife and some imagination.

- Always garnish food at the last minute to keep it looking fresh and inviting.

- Before garnishing dishes that have been standing or refrigerated, give them a gentle stir bringing the dressing, juices or marinade to the surface. This gives the food an inviting sheen.

- Easy garnishes include:

    julienned vegetables

    whole leaves or sprigs of herbs

    finely minced peppers or herbs thrown confetti style onto the plate

    fresh grated cheese

    thin rings of red onion or peppers

    slices of lemons, limes, pineapples or oranges

    snipped chives or scallion greens

    quartered cherry or plum tomatoes

    crisp celery leaves

    dollops of fat-free sour cream dusted with paprika or red pepper

- Give fresh herb leaves pizzazz by dipping them into cold water, shaking off the excess, then dipping leaf edges in paprika.

- Make a fruit or vegetable twist by taking a thin, round slice of orange, lemon or cucumber; make one cut from the center to the edge; then twist the slice in opposite directions into a spiral or S shape so the round will stand upright when placed on the dish.

- Make scallion brushes by trimming the root end of a scallion; then, using a sharp, pointed knife, slash both ends thin at one-eighth-inch intervals. Leave an inch uncut in the center of the scallion. Place in a bowl of ice water, and the slashed tips will curl within fifteen minutes.

- Fan out fruits and vegetables by cutting them lengthwise into thin slices with a sharp, pointed knife. Cut to within one-fourth inch of the stem end. Use your fingers to fan out the fruit or vegetable.

- Make a chiffonade of greens to garnish rice, vegetables or meat by stacking the leaves of greens such as romaine, green or red leaf lettuce, or spinach; roll them into a cigar shape; then thinly slice crosswise. The resulting "ribbons" of green make a garnish that's both flavorful and colorful.

- Make a radish rose by using a sharp knife to cut thin petals of the red peel vertically around the radish from the tip down almost to the stem end. Put radishes in a bowl of ice water, cover and refrigerate for an hour, or until petals pull away from the center portion.

How the Menus and Recipes Work

On the following pages are menus that incorporate all of my principles for great food and great health. Each menu is made up of separate recipes that have been designed to form a pleasing whole of contrasting tastes, textures and colors.

Each recipe grouping is arbitrary, influenced by such factors as market availability and personal food preferences. Use my menus as points of departure. Reorganize as you wish, taking a recipe from one menu and adding it to another, or substitute ingredients if you are missing one. You can use the foods you have on hand to create something new and personally yours.

Planning Your Plate

The breakfast, lunch and dinner sections of *Healthy Living* have been designed using a whole meal approach. Rather than ten chicken recipes, five beef recipes and so on, I show you how to serve up complete meals that give taste, beauty in presentation and nutritional balance.

Each meal begins with a breakdown of the meal's source of protein, complex carbohydrate and simple carbohydrate. Sometimes the recipe for that nutrient source will be included for you;

at other times it will be an easy add-on source of nutrition, like a simple glass of skim milk.

A healthy meal consists of larger amounts of carbohydrates and smaller amounts of protein than you may have eaten in the past. Generally, a single serving of a lunch or dinner main dish will give a maximum of three to four ounces of protein, a far cry from the sixteen-ounce steaks we feasted on when we were growing up!

Protein should be part of the meal but not its focus. As critical as protein is to our wellness in building up the body, we need smaller amounts of it spread more evenly throughout the day, rather than a hunk of meat overloaded into one huge meal.

A Word About Nutritional Profile Charts

Per Serving: Calories

Protein gr.	Carb. gr.
Fat gr.	Cal. from fat %
Chol. mg.	Sodium mg.

With the help of my computer I have analyzed each recipe in *Healthy Living* for its nutritional value. Besides the calories and the carbohydrate, protein and fat grams, I have included information about sodium and cholesterol for those of you who are watching these numbers as well. The fat grams are also expressed in terms of the percentage of calories derived from fat in each particular dish. My meals are designed to give less than 25 percent of the calories from fat, with the average dish yielding 17 percent. Individual recipes that may be higher in percentage of fat calories are paired with those having low or no fat to balance the whole meal properly.

The nutrient values listed are as accurate as possible and are based on certain assumptions:

- All nutrient breakdowns are listed per serving.

- All meats are trimmed of all visible fat and skin before cooking.

- When a range is given for an ingredient (for example, one to two teaspoons), the

good cooking

lesser amount is calculated.

- When an option is given for ingredients, the first option is calculated.

- A large percentage of calories from alcohol evaporates in cooking, and this is reflected in the profiles.

- When a marinade is used, only the amount absorbed into the food is calculated.

- Garnishes and optional ingredients are not calculated.

Please note also that the analysis is for the recipe ingredients only. Many times you will see a dotted line underneath the ingredients followed by a note that says, "Serve with…" This note may tell you that Strawberry Sauce, Black Bean and Corn Salsa or some other dish is to be served with that meal, though the complete recipe is not shown. The "serve with" items will not be included in the nutritional analysis for that recipe. You may look up the nutritional analysis for the sauce or salsa on the page where their complete recipes are shown.

I have used these profiles to plan balanced meals that give appropriate levels of nutrients. Portion sizes may need to be adjusted to fit caloric needs according to your own individual meal plan. Calorie requirements will vary according to your age, size, weight, level of activity and even stress levels. So don't get caught up in counting every calorie you eat. Instead, focus on eating great foods, prepared in great ways, that are great for you.

Meal-Planning Tips

- **Go for color.** Go for blueberries, raspberries, mango, papaya, watermelon, honeydew, cantaloupe, apple, orange or grapefruit. Go for broccoli, tomatoes, spinach, romaine lettuce, sweet potatoes and carrots. Have a minimum of five servings of fruits or vegetables each day—ideally nine to ten servings!

- **Go for grains.** Whole grains provide fiber and help stabilize blood sugar levels for several hours after eating. Vary your breads—try whole-grain English muffins, pita pockets, tortillas or rolls. Choose oats, brown rice or whole-wheat pasta when possible, and experiment with spelt, barley, quinoa, cracked wheat, wild rice and whole-grain couscous.

- **Eat beans five or more times a week.** Legumes are one of the highest-fiber foods you can find. Beans are especially high in soluble fiber, which lowers cholesterol levels, and folate, which lowers levels of homocysteine, another risk factor for heart disease. (Quick tip: To reduce sodium in canned beans by about one-third, rinse off the canning liquid before using. Or look for canned beans with no added sodium.) Jazz them up with liberal use of garlic and hot peppers for added nutraceutical punch. Also try Black Bean Dip (page 61) and other bean spreads—they make great snacks with whole-grain crackers or baked tortilla chips.

- **Have a soy food every day.** This could be soy milk, soy cheese, tofu, soy nuts, a veggie burger, tempeh or soy protein isolate powder added to a power shake.

- **Eat fish at least twice a week.** To get the most omega-3s, choose salmon, canned white albacore tuna in water, rainbow trout, anchovies, herring, sardines and mackerel. Or get a plant version of omega-3 fat in flaxseed.

- **Eat nuts five times a week.** Learn to incorporate these luscious morsels into your diet almost every day. The key to eating nuts healthfully is not to eat too many—they're so high in calories that you could easily *gain* weight. To help avoid temptation, keep nuts in your fridge—where they are safe from oxidizing and turning rancid and where they are out of sight. Sprinkle 2 tablespoons a day on cereal, yogurt, veggies, salads or wherever the crunch and rich flavor appeal to you, or have Trail Mix as a frequent Power Snack.

If you struggle to eat well, you are more than likely among the nutrient-deficient majority—and you aren't getting what it takes to live fit and fueled. Here's the bottom line: We will only eat well and cook well if we fill our pantries with the right foods. Unhealthy food traps can be avoided if they are out of sight and out of mind—then they will be out of mouth. Rethinking your food supply is a major step toward making healthy habits. Eating well is much simpler if nutritious foods are kept within reach.

good cooking

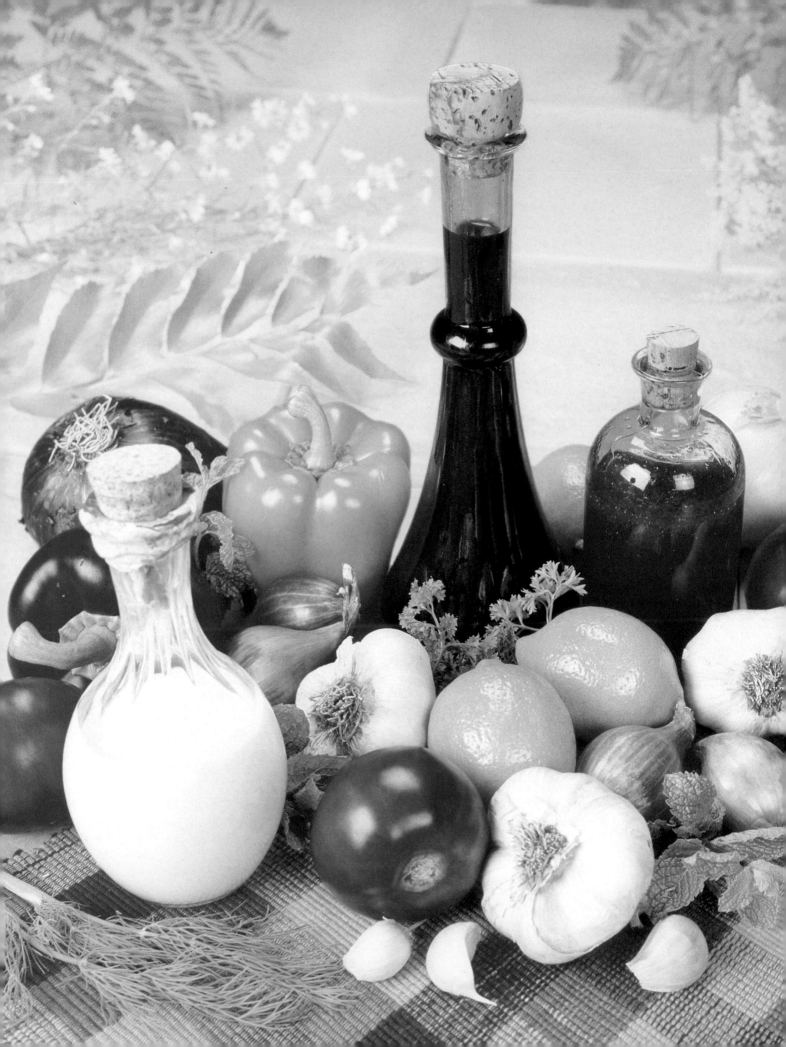

the well-stocked kitchen

TIPS & RECIPES

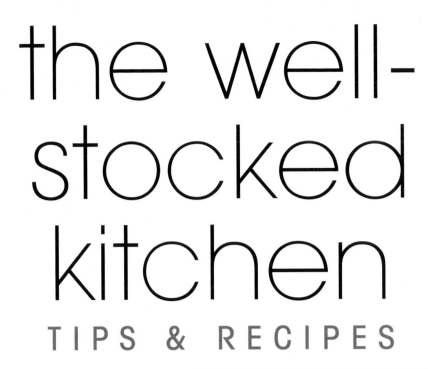

Food shopping today in the United States offers more healthy possibilities than ever before. You have choices, and I encourage you to search out the best. Great meals begin with the best-quality ingredients.

A well-stocked kitchen makes the difference between efficiently putting together healthy, flavorful foods vs. a meal-time-blues headache or a fast-food nightmare.

Smart Shopping Tips

PICK THE BEST SHOP FOR THE JOB: From artisan bakeries and ethnic-food markets to well-stocked supermarkets and natural food stores—find out where you can get the best product. Where can you get the freshest fish? Where can you get the best-tasting 100 percent, whole-grain breads and baked goods? It may mean an extra trip once a week, or even once a month—so stock up your freezer with the goods.

Pictured: Fresh ingredients for healthy cooking

ALWAYS SHOP WITH A LIST: I know you know this—but whether you shop once a week or several times a week, a list is essential for efficiency and to help you cut back on impulse buying. And don't shop hungry!

Once you've planned your menus, begin your list by writing down all the ingredients you'll need. Then "shop" your refrigerator, freezer and pantry first. Cross off the list those ingredients you already have. Then head to the market for the rest.

I try to shop once a month to restock my pantry with nonperishable items and my freezer with those I can store there. Then I can quickly shop a few times a week just to pick up the fresh foods.

GET TO KNOW SHOPKEEPERS AND MANAGERS: If you primarily shop at supermarkets,

the well-stocked kitchen

Whole-Grain Cereal Choices:

- *All Bran With Extra Fiber*

- *Cheerios*

- *Familia Müesli Granola (no sugar added)*

- *Grape-Nuts*

- *Kashi*

- *Kellogg's Just Right*

- *Kellogg's Nutri-Grain (wheat, corn or almond raisin)*

- *Kellogg's Raisin Squares*

- *Nabisco Shredded Wheat*

- *Post Bran Flakes*

- *Ralston Muesli*

get to know the managers of the produce, meat and seafood departments. Find out the days they are most apt to get the best deliveries of which products—and shop on those days. And don't be afraid to ask your new friends to carry a new product you have heard about or to special order just for you.

AFTER YOU'VE SHOPPED: Plan to use the most perishable foods first (fresh seafood, leafy vegetables, fresh berries and stone fruits). Saving the hardiest foods for last (carrots, broccoli, apples, meats) will help reduce waste and eliminate unnecessary trips to the store.

Choosing Cereal, Breads and Grains

Whole grain is a must for fiber and nutrition. The word *whole* should be the first word of the ingredient list, such as "whole wheat, whole oats." Also check labels for hidden fats and hidden sugars; some cereals, like granola, are nutritional nightmares in a bowl. Cereals should have less than 5 grams of added sugar, excluding that from any dried fruit it may contain.

Look for a variety of whole-grain English muffins, small-size bagels, tortillas, pitas and crackers—your natural food store is most apt to have 100 percent whole-grain choices. Remember the available variety of whole-grain English muffins, bagels, pita breads and, of course, rice cakes.

Buying the Basics

Stock up on whole-wheat or artichoke pastas and brown rice—they are chewier and more filling than their white-flour counterparts and are a nice alternative. Also go for other grains such as amaranth, barley, cracked wheat, whole-wheat couscous, quinoa and spelt.

Include dried or canned beans, split peas, lentils and chickpeas.

Daring Dairy

Although they get a bad rap these days, dairy foods are a treasure chest of protein, calcium and other body-building nutrients. But they can also be loaded with fat, so look for lower-fat variations on favorites: skim milk, buttermilk, nonfat yogurt, skim-milk ricotta, pot or farmer's cheese, part-skim mozzarella and skim-milk cottage cheese. Check the labels to be sure they fit your nutrition standards of having fewer than 3 grams of fat per 100-calorie serving.

Doing the Deli

Select sliced turkey or chicken, lean ham and low-fat cheeses instead of the usual lunch meats. Limit use of high-fat, high-sodium processed sausages and meats, hot dogs, bacon and salami.

Fending Against Fats and Oils

I use small amounts of healthy and flavorful monounsaturated extra-virgin olive oil for most all of my cooking—flavorless canola and grapeseed oil for the occasional recipe that doesn't fare well with the flavor of olive oil. I also use a drizzle of flavorful sesame oil and walnut oil for certain special recipes—but never for cooking; they do not stand up well to heat.

Oils should be purchased in small bottles and kept tightly closed in a cool, dimly lit spot in your kitchen or pantry. Exposure to light and air oxidizes the oils.

If I have to make a choice between butter or margarine, I always choose limited amounts of a real food—butter. Buy good quality butter and keep it frozen. Avoid hydrogenated fat and trans fats whenever possible—label reading is a must here. Similarly, I vote for reduced-fat or light mayonnaise or dressings—not fat free, which are often just chemical brews loaded with sugars.

Finding Fish

I strongly recommend fish and seafood as a source of protein and for the healthy type of fat it provides. Virtually all fish contains some heart-protective, health-enhancing omega-3 fatty acids, and population studies around the world show health benefits from eating fish of all kinds. I plan my weekly meals to include three to four servings. The fish with the most omega-3 fatty acids are oily, cold-water varieties like salmon, trout, tuna, mackerel and sardines.

About fish safety: There is no other type of food in which freshness and purity is so critical. Know your "fishmonger," find out when the fish comes in, and buy on those days. Really fresh seafood should smell faintly of the sea, but sweet. It should not be offensively rank or have a "fishy," ammonia-like smell.

Because almost all shrimp has been frozen when caught, I ask for two- or five-pound bags, still frozen, and defrost only what I need, when I need it.

Knowing Nuts

Nuts and seeds, although a source of fat, are wonderfully nutritious additions to your pantry. Use sparingly and take care with buying and storing them. As with most healthy ingredients, fresh is king—the naturally occurring oils in nuts and seeds can quickly go rancid.

Buy only fresh nuts and seeds, store them tightly covered in the refrigerator or freezer, and check them regularly for freshness. Rancidity is usually detectable by your nose or taste buds—sniff first, and throw out any products that develop an off smell.

Seeking Soy Foods

Soy milk can now be found in the dairy case, as well as in shelf-stable boxes. Firm and soft tofu is available in refrigerated tubs in the produce section and in shelf-stable boxes on the grocer's shelves. Edamame (green soybeans in their pods) and already-shelled "sweet beans" make a great side dish and fun-to-eat appetizer or snack. Look for them in the frozen-food section. And tempeh—a tender, chunky soybean cake—is commonly available in the freezer section of a natural food store.

Making Meat Choices

All cuts should be lean and trimmed of visible fat. Choose the following: beef—round, loin, sirloin and extra-lean ground beef; lamb—leg, arm, loin, rib; pork— tenderloin, leg, shoulder; turkey or chicken—skinless; fish and shellfish— fresh, just delivered.

Water, Water Everywhere

Stock up on bottled waters to replace sugary sodas, which offer zero nutrition and lots of calories. Try sparkling mineral waters (add a splash of fruit juice for flavor).

Picking Produce

Fruits and vegetables are no-fat, no-cholesterol beauties with fiber that help in stabilizing the body—providing for lower cholesterol levels, boosted immunities against sicknesses, lovelier skin, nails and hair, higher energy levels and less body aches and pains. Keep enough on hand so that you can always make a salad. Buy the freshest—and the most colorful—produce possible for top nutrition. Generally, the more vivid the coloring of the pulp, the more essential nutrients it holds.

Wonderfully fresh fruits and vegetables are a particular passion of mine. For the sweetest produce, choose what is in season—a good price and abundant supply will tell you a fruit or vegetable is at its peak. Ask at your grocery store or farmer's market which are freshest buying days and where the vegetables are grown; search for locally grown and in-season fruits and vegetables. Out-of-season produce is more expensive and often imported. If it is imported, it may be only spot-checked for pesticide residues. (Use the fruit and vegetable guides on pages 38 through 41 when getting ready to purchase fruit or vegetables.)

When fresh is not possible, frozen is the next choice; avoid vegetables that are prepared with butters or sauces, and fruits that are packed with sugar. (Freezing foods doesn't destroy their nutrients and quality as readily as canning does.)

Take advantage of your grocer's pre-cut, pre-chopped vegetables and fruits. They are available in the produce area or may be purchased by the pound from the salad bar.

the well-stocked kitchen

A Guide to Sweet and Wonderful Fruit

Fruit	Description	Serving Size
Apples	Should be firm and crisp without a watery, soft give. Excellent for eating: Braeburn, Red and Golden Delicious, Elstar, Fuji, Granny Smith, McIntosh, Jonathan, Winesap. Excellent for cooking: Golden Delicious, Rome Beauty, Cortland, Granny Smith, McIntosh (never Red Delicious as they are too dry). Hint: Drizzling cut apples with lemon juice will prevent browning.	1 small apple
Apricots	Should be fat and golden. Easiest to find in dried form. Very high in potassium and vitamin A.	2 fresh or 4 dried halves
Avocados	Use sparingly since avocados are a source of fat. They are ripe when soft to the touch and skin is darkened.	⅛ whole or 2 Tbsp. mashed avocado
Bananas	Are considered ripe when covered with brown specks. Once ripe, refrigeration will keep them in excellent eating condition for another three to five days. (Skin may brown completely.) Bananas are very high in potassium. They are best for use as a sweetener when very brown and ripe. Hint: If using in fruit salad, top the salad with sliced bananas just before serving and sprinkle with lemon juice to prevent browning.	½ large or 1 small (6-inch) banana
Berries	Sweet packages of nutritional power. Berries should be firm when purchased; avoid stained containers.	½ cup
Cantaloupe	Very high in vitamins A and C; also potassium. The outside should be dull, creamy yellow when purchased, and the blossom end should be slightly soft when ripe. Look for pronounced lacy netting.	¼ cantaloupe or ¾ cup cubed
Coconut	Use sparingly since it is a source of fat. Most natural food stores have unsweetened flaked coconut. For fresher flavor, soak in small amount of milk before cooking.	2 Tbsp. unsweetened flaked coconut
Figs	Should be ripe (soft when squeezed) and plump; should smell sweet, not sour. Refrigerate.	1 medium fig
Grapefruit and oranges	Should be round, heavy for their size and thin-skinned.	½ grapefruit 1 medium orange ½ cup sections
Grapes	Choose a ripe bunch. Do not ripen off the vine. The point where the grape attaches to stem should be strong and fresh, and grapes should have a full color.	12 grapes

Fruit	Description	Serving Size
Honeydew	Should have a soft blossom end; skin should be slightly sticky.	1/8 honeydew
Kiwi	Should yield slightly to the touch.	1 kiwi
Mangoes	Should yield slightly to the touch but should not be soft.	1/3 whole or 1/3 cup diced
Nectarines, peaches and pears	Are ripe when slightly soft at stem end and yellowish rather than greenish. Peaches and nectarines should have a pink blush as well. To help with the ripening, place nectarines, peaches, pears or plums in a brown paper bag with a banana. As the banana ripens, it releases a natural gas that ripens the other fruit as if still on the tree.	1 medium fruit
Papaya	Should be mostly yellow, should yield slightly to pressure and have a pleasant aroma.	3/4 cup cubed
Pineapple	Is ripe when it has deep green leaves at the crown, heaviness for its size and a sweet aroma (not fermented or acidic). It should yield slightly when pressed with finger.	2 slices or 1/3 cup chunked or crushed
Plums	Should not be rock hard but plump and firm to the touch.	2 small plums
Watermelon	Should be purchased with a smooth surface, dullish sheen and a creamy yellow underside.	1 cup cubed melon

Dried Fruit

Fruit	Serving Size
Dried apple rings	1/2 ounce or 8 rings
Dried apricots	4 halves
Dates (unsweetened)	2 dates
Dried peaches, pears	1 fruit
Prunes	2 large prunes
Raisins	2 Tbsp. or 1 small box

A Guide to Vibrant Vegetables

Vegetable	Preparation	Minutes to Steam	Yield	Complementary Seasonings
Asparagus	remove tough ends before cooking; stand in boiling water	5 minutes uncovered, then 7 to 10 minutes covered	1 lb. raw = 2 cups cooked	chives, garlic, lemon juice, parsley
Green beans	wash and snap ends off	8 to 10 minutes until crisp tender	1 lb. raw = 3 cups cooked	basil, dill, garlic, lemon, parsley, rosemary
Beets	scrub well; do not peel	20 to 30 minutes until crisp tender	1 lb. raw = 3 cups cooked	basil, cloves, mint, tarragon
Broccoli	pare stalk of tough skin before cooking	8 to 20 minutes until crisp tender	1 bunch (2 lbs.) raw = 2 cups cooked	garlic, lemon juice, pimento, vinegar
Brussels sprouts	cut off stems and slash stem ends for quicker cooking	12 minutes	1 lb. raw = 3 cups cooked	chives, nutmeg
Cabbage	core and cut into wedges or quarters or shred	12 to 15 minutes for wedges; 5 minutes for shredded	1 lb. raw = 2 cups cooked	basil, caraway seeds, dill, poppy seeds, sage
Carrots	scrub thoroughly or pare; leave whole or slice	10 minutes	7 to 8 raw = 2 cups cooked	basil, ginger, mint, nutmeg, parsley
Cauliflower	core and remove outer leaves; leave whole or cut into florets	12 to 15 minutes	1 head (2 lbs.) raw = 3 cups cooked	basil, chives, nutmeg, rosemary, tarragon
Corn	remove husks; remove silk; wash	boil or steam for 8 minutes	1 small ear = ½ cup	celery seeds, chives, green pepper, pimento
Eggplant	peel and slice; salt slices and let stand 15 minutes; rinse well before use	better to grill 5 to 7 minutes or use in soups or casseroles	11 slices (½-inch thick) raw = 2 cups cooked	basil, oregano, parsley, tarragon, thyme
Greens	wash well; discard discolored leaves	8 to 9 minutes or until wilted	1 lb. raw = 1½ to 2 cups cooked	basil, dill, oregano, onion, black pepper, vinegar
Mushrooms	wash gently or wipe with damp cloth; trim stem ends	sauté for 5 to 7 minutes or use raw or cooked in other dishes	10 mushrooms raw = 1 cup cooked	basil, chives, marjoram, parsley, thyme

Vegetable	Preparation	Minutes to Steam	Yield	Complementary Seasonings
Okra	wash and remove stem ends	use in mixtures for soups and stews	1 lb. raw = 2 cups cooked	basil, bay leaf, onion, parsley, thyme
Onions	remove outer, loosest layer of skin	sauté 3 to 4 minutes or bake at 400 degrees for 40 minutes	1 medium = ½ cup chopped	dill, cloves, mint, parsley, tarragon
Parsnips	scrub well or pare; leave whole or slice	10 minutes	4 medium raw = 1 cup cooked	dill, parsley, sage
Peas	shell and wash	6 to 7 minutes	1 lb. raw = 1 cup cooked	basil, dill, mint, parsley, rosemary
Potatoes, white and sweet	scrub and remove any brown spots; do not peel	bake 1 hour; steam 15 to 20 minutes	3 medium raw = 2½ cups cooked	white: dill, chives, parsley, rosemary sweet: chives, cinnamon, nutmeg
Spinach	wash thoroughly and remove stems; serve raw in salads	steam 4 to 5 minutes until wilted	1 lb. raw = 1½ to 2 cups cooked	basil, chives, dill, garlic, lemon, vinegar
Squash, spaghetti	cut in half; remove seeds and place cut side down in small amount of water on a baking sheet	bake at 350 degrees for 45 minutes, until strands pull free with a fork	1 squash (2 lbs.) = 2 cups cooked	basil, oregano, parsley
Squash, summer	wash; trim off ends	steam or boil for 6 to 8 minutes	2 lbs. raw = 2 cups cooked	basil, oregano, parsley
Squash, winter	wash; cut in half and place cut side down on baking sheet, or peel and cut into small pieces to steam	bake at 350 degrees for 1 hour or steam pieces for 20 to 30 minutes	2 lbs. raw = 2 cups cooked	cinnamon, nutmeg, orange peel

Pam Smith's
Healthy Living Grocery List

GRAINS AND BREADS
☐ Barley
Brown rice: ☐ Instant
    ☐ Long-grain ☐ Short-grain
    ☐ Wild rice ☐ Arborio rice
☐ Cornmeal
☐ Couscous
Tortillas, flour: ☐ Mission
    ☐ Buena Vida Fat Free
☐ Whole-wheat bagels
☐ 100% whole-wheat bread
    ("whole" is the first word of the
    ingredients)
☐ Whole-wheat English muffins
☐ Whole-wheat hamburger buns
Whole-wheat or artichoke pasta:
    ☐ Angel hair ☐ Elbows
    ☐ Flat ☐ Orzo ☐ Lasagna
    ☐ Penne ☐ Spaghetti
    ☐ Rotini (spirals)
☐ Whole-wheat pastry flour
☐ Whole-wheat pita bread
☐ _____
☐ _____

CEREALS (whole-grain and less
than 5 grams of added sugar):
☐ All Bran With Extra Fiber
☐ Bran Buds
☐ Cheerios
☐ Familia Müesli
☐ Grape-Nuts
☐ Grits ☐ Kashi
☐ Kellogg's Just Right
☐ Kellogg's Low Fat Granola
☐ Kellogg's Raisin Squares
☐ Nabisco Shredded Wheat
☐ Ralston Muesli
Oats: ☐ Old-fashioned
    ☐ Quick-cooking
☐ Post Bran Flakes
Puffed cereals: ☐ Rice ☐ Wheat
☐ Shredded Wheat 'N Bran
Unprocessed bran: ☐ Oat
    ☐ Wheat ☐ Rice
☐ Wheatena
☐ _____

CRACKERS
Crispbread: ☐ Kavli ☐ Wasa
☐ Crispy cakes
☐ Health Valley graham crackers
☐ Harvest Crisps 5-Grain (not all
    whole grain, but good for variety)
Rice Cakes: ☐ Plain
    ☐ Quaker Banana Nut
☐ Ry Vita Whole-grain Crispbread
☐ Ry Krisp
☐ _____
☐ _____

DAIRY
☐ Butter ☐ Light butter
Cheese (low-fat—fewer than
    5 grams of fat per ounce):
    Cheddar:
      ☐ Kraft Fat Free
      ☐ Kraft Natural Reduced Fat
    ☐ Cottage cheese (1% or nonfat)
    Cream cheese:
      ☐ Philadelphia Light (tub)
      ☐ Philadelphia Free
    ☐ Farmer's
    ☐ Jarlsberg Lite
    Mozzarella: ☐ Nonfat
      ☐ Part-skim
      ☐ String cheese
    Nonrefrigerated:
      ☐ Laughing Cow Light
    ☐ Parmesan
    Ricotta: ☐ Nonfat ☐ Skim milk
      ☐ Sun-Ni Armenian String
☐ Egg substitute
☐ Eggs
☐ Milk (skim or 1%)
☐ Nonfat sour cream
☐ Nonfat plain yogurt
☐ Stonyfield Farm yogurt
☐ Silk (soy milk)
☐ Veggie-Slices (Tofu Cheese)

CANNED GOODS
Chicken broth: ☐ Swanson's
    Natural Goodness
☐ Evaporated skim milk

☐ Hearts of Palm
Soups: ☐ Healthy Choice
    ☐ Pritikin
    ☐ Progresso Hearty Black Bean
    ☐ Progresso Lentil
Tomatoes: ☐ Fresh Cut ☐ Paste
    ☐ Sauce ☐ Stewed ☐ Whole
☐ _____
☐ _____
☐ _____

CONDIMENTS
☐ Honey
Hot Pepper Sauce:
    ☐ Pickapeppa sauce
    ☐ Shriracha Chili Sauce
    ☐ Jamaican Hell Fire
    ☐ Tabasco
Mayonnaise: ☐ Light
    ☐ Miracle Whip Light
Mustard: ☐ Dijon ☐ Spicy hot
☐ Pepperoncini peppers
Salad Dressing:
    ☐ Bernstein's Reduced Calorie
    ☐ Good Seasons ☐ Kraft Free
    ☐ Jardine's Fat Free Garlic
      Vinaigrette
    ☐ Pritikin
☐ Soy sauce (low-sodium)
☐ Salsa or picante sauce
Spices and herbs: ☐ Allspice
    ☐ Basil ☐ Black pepper
    ☐ Cayenne ☐ Celery seed
    ☐ Chili powder ☐ Cinnamon
    ☐ Creole seasoning ☐ Curry
    ☐ Dill weed ☐ Five spice
    ☐ Garlic powder ☐ Ginger
    ☐ Mrs. Dash Original Blend
    ☐ Mrs. Dash Garlic and Herb
      Seasoning
    ☐ Mustard ☐ Nutmeg
    ☐ Oregano
    ☐ Onion powder
    ☐ Paprika ☐ Parsley
    ☐ Pepper, cracked
    ☐ Rosemary ☐ Saffron
    ☐ Salt ☐ Thyme

Fresh herbs: ☐ Basil
    ☐ Chives ☐ Cilantro ☐ Ginger
    ☐ Parsley ☐ Rosemary ☐ Thyme
☐ Vanilla extract
Vinegars: ☐ Balsamic ☐ Cider
    ☐ Red wine ☐ Rice wine
    ☐ Tarragon ☐ White wine
☐ Lea and Perrins Worcestershire
    for Chicken
☐ _____

FRUITS

Fresh fruits: ☐ Apples ☐ Apricots
    ☐ Bananas ☐ Berries ☐ Cherries
    ☐ Dates (unsweetened, pitted)
    ☐ Grapefruit ☐ Grapes ☐ Kiwi
    ☐ Lemons ☐ Limes ☐ Mango
    ☐ Melon ☐ Nectarines
    ☐ Oranges ☐ Papaya ☐ Peaches
    ☐ Pears ☐ Pineapple ☐ Plantains
    ☐ Plums
Dried fruits: ☐ Apricots ☐ Craisins
    ☐ Peaches ☐ Pineapple
    ☐ Raisins (dark and golden)
    ☐ Mixed
☐ _____
☐ _____

VEGETABLES

☐ Asparagus   ☐ Beets
☐ Bell peppers   ☐ Broccoli
☐ Brussels sprouts ☐ Cabbage
☐ Carrots ☐ Cauliflower ☐ Celery
☐ Corn ☐ Cucumbers ☐ Eggplant
☐ Garlic ☐ Green beans ☐ Greens
☐ Hot peppers ☐ Kale
☐ Mushrooms ☐ Okra ☐ Onions
☐ Peas ☐ Red potatoes ☐ Radicchio
☐ Romaine lettuce
☐ Salad greens ☐ Shallots
☐ Simply Potatoes hash browns
☐ Spinach
☐ Squash (yellow, crookneck)
☐ Sugar snap peas (frozen)
☐ Sun-dried tomatoes
☐ Sweet potatoes ☐ Tomatoes
☐ White potatoes ☐ Zucchini
☐ _____
☐ _____
☐ _____
☐ _____
☐ _____

BEANS AND MEATS

Beans and peas: ☐ Black
    ☐ Chickpeas/garbanzo beans
    ☐ Cannelini ☐ Kidney ☐ Lentils
    ☐ Navy ☐ Pinto ☐ Split peas
Beef (lean):
    ☐ Deli-sliced
    ☐ Ground round
    ☐ London broil
    ☐ Round steak
Fish and seafood:
    ☐ Clams   ☐ Cod
    ☐ Grouper   ☐ Mussels
    ☐ Salmon   ☐ Scallops
    ☐ Shrimp   ☐ Snapper
    ☐ Swordfish   ☐ Tuna
☐ Garden Burger
Lamb: ☐ Leg   ☐ Loin chops
Pork: ☐ Canadian bacon
    ☐ Center-cut chops
    ☐ Tenderloin
Poultry:
    Chicken: ☐ Boneless breasts
    ☐ Legs/thighs
    ☐ Whole fryer
    Turkey: ☐ Bacon ☐ Breast
    ☐ Ground extra lean
    ☐ Deli-sliced
    ☐ Whole
    ☐ _____
    ☐ _____
Soy: ☐ Boca Burgers ☐ Tofu
    ☐ Tempeh
Veal: ☐ Chops ☐ Cutlets
    ☐ Ground
Water-packed cans: ☐ Chicken
    ☐ Salmon ☐ Tuna
    ☐ Charlie's Lunch Kit
☐ _____
☐ _____
☐ _____

MISCELLANEOUS

All-fruit spreads and pourable fruit: .
    ☐ Knudsen   ☐ Polaner
    ☐ Smucker's Simply Fruit
    ☐ Welch's Totally Fruit
☐ Baking powder
☐ Baking soda
Bean dips (Fat-free): ☐ Jardine's
    ☐ Guiltless Gourmet
☐ Bread crumbs

Cooking oils: ☐ Canola ☐ Olive
☐ Cornstarch
Fruit Juices (unsweetened):
    ☐ Apple   ☐ Cranberry-apple
    ☐ White grape ☐ Orange
☐ Nonstick cooking spray
Nuts/seeds (dry-roasted, unsalted):
    ☐ Flaxseed ☐ Peanuts ☐ Pecans
    ☐ Pumpkin Seeds ☐ Soynuts
    ☐ Sunflower kernels
    ☐ Walnuts
Pasta Sauce: ☐ Pritikin
    ☐ Classico Tomato and Basil
    ☐ Ragu Chunky Gardenstyle
☐ Peanut butter (natural)
☐ Phyllo dough
☐ Popcorn—Orville Redenbacher's
    Natural Light or Smart Pop
    microwave popcorn
☐ Plain kernels
☐ _____
Tortilla chips: ☐ Baked Tostitos
    ☐ Guiltless Gourmet
☐ Water (spring or sparkling)
Wine: ☐ Dealcoholized
    ☐ Red ☐ White
☐ _____
☐ _____
☐ _____
☐ _____
☐ _____
☐ _____
☐ _____
☐ _____
☐ _____
☐ _____
☐ _____
☐ _____
☐ _____
☐ _____
☐ _____
☐ _____
☐ _____
☐ _____
☐ _____
☐ _____

the well-stocked kitchen

Homemade Creole Seasoning

Prepare the following recipe for homemade creole seasoning, and store it in an airtight container, ready to add to your favorite recipe:

Homemade Creole Seasoning

2 1/2 Tbsp. paprika
2 Tbsp. garlic powder
1 Tbsp. salt
1 Tbsp. onion powder
1 Tbsp. dried oregano
1 Tbsp. dried thyme
1 Tbsp. red pepper
1 Tbsp. black pepper

Combine all ingredients in a small bowl; stir well. Store in an airtight container. Yield: about 2/3 cup (serving size: 1 tsp.)

1 tsp. gives 201 mg. sodium.

Special Grocery Items

A few of the ingredients used in the *Healthy Living* grocery list and recipes may be unfamiliar to you or may not be available at your local supermarket, depending on the region. Ask your grocer for help, or try a nearby health food store or ethnic specialty shop.

ARBORIO RICE: This Italian grain is a must for risotto because the high-starch kernels add creamy texture. Arborio is now found in most supermarket and health food stores.

ARUGULA: This aromatic green lends a special flavor to salads. It is sold in small bunches in the supermarket produce section or farmer's markets.

CANADIAN BACON: The lean eye meat of a pork loin, this low-fat breakfast meat is not just for breakfast. Adding 1 to 2 tablespoons of finely chopped Canadian bacon at the end of cooking any recipe calling for salt pork or bacon will yield a delicious, smoky presence with far less fat. Use it occasionally, and enjoy it!

CAPERS: These little packages of flavor pack a powerful punch—sour, bitter and salty all at the same time. You'll find them in the supermarket's condiment section pickled and packed in small jars. You'll use them sparingly because they are so highly salted, never more than 1 tablespoon in a serving. Always rinse capers before using. Don't despair using such a small amount; they last in the refrigerator for several weeks.

CILANTRO: The flat leaf of the coriander plant, this herb is also called Chinese parsley and fresh coriander. It's terrific in Mexican, Asian and Caribbean dishes, but if it's new to you, use it sparingly (start with just a teaspoon): Too much can make the dish taste like soap! You'll find it looking like parsley in the produce department of the supermarket.

COUSCOUS: These tiny beads of ground wheat semolina resemble rice, but couscous is actually a type of pasta. Most couscous you find will be precooked; it requires only a 5-minute plumping in hot stock or water. Whole-wheat couscous is available at health food stores.

CREOLE SEASONING: The blend of spices used in creole seasonings can add a sassy surprise to your favorite recipes for soups, meat dishes and salads. Make your own creole seasoning, and keep it handy when you cook. Or you can purchase it in the spice aisle.
Tony Chachere's is my favorite!

EVAPORATED SKIM MILK: This is a terrific way to add richness and creaminess to a sauce without heavy cream. It has a creamlike flavor and is richer in texture than regular milk. You'll find it in the baking ingredients aisle of the supermarket with the shelf-stable milks such as Parmalat— another new milk that's great to keep on hand and to travel with.

EUROPEAN CUCUMBERS: You'll find these long, dark green cucumbers vacuum-seal-wrapped in the produce department. Their claim to fame is that they are seedless and crisp—and don't bring on the indigestion of their "normal" cucumber cousins.

FISH SAUCE: This is an essential Asian ingredient and can be used in place of soy sauce. The better brands are really wonderful. Look for it packaged in glass, not plastic, from companies in Thailand.

FIVE SPICE: Chinese five spice powder is a blend of equal parts of cinnamon, cloves, fennel seed, star anise and Szechuan peppercorns. It has a pungent, slightly sweet licorice flavor and is used in Oriental cuisine.

FRUIT JUICES: 100 percent pure juices (no sugar added) make wonderful marinades, bringing out the flavor of foods such as poultry and seafood. In their concentrated form they are also natural sweeteners that can easily replace refined sugar.

SALAD GREENS: There are many exotic greens found in the salads of *Healthy Living*— frizee, radicchio and arugula among them. Ask your produce grocer about their availability; they add much interest to a salad. If you don't have these, substitute red leaf lettuce along with romaine and green leaf lettuces.

HERBS: These are surprise packages of flavor—accenting and enhancing the flavor of whatever you serve. Whole leaves of basil, cilantro, thyme and rosemary are wonderful for garnish; a chopped mixture is great to throw into a dish while cooking and onto the whole plate confetti-style when serving.

You may also use dried herbs in cooking and save the fresh herbs for garnish where their full flavor can be enjoyed. Because dried herbs are so much stronger than fresh, use only one-third as much (1 tablespoon of fresh equals 1 teaspoon of dried).

Finely chop and blend the following herbs: 1 bunch cilantro, 1 bunch basil, 1 bunch rosemary and 1 bunch thyme. You may store them in your refrigerator for several days. Add them as you prepare your favorite recipes.

To wash herbs, fill a pitcher with water, and hold herbs by the stem while swishing them in the water. Lay them on paper towels to dry.

ORZO: This tiny pasta resembles a soft, wonderful rice. Orzo cooks up in about five minutes and makes a delightful side dish.

PARMESAN CHEESE: Don't even bother with the pre-grated Parmesan cheese dust — it's not worth the fat calories. But do try a chunk of fresh Parmesan grated directly onto your meals right as you're serving. The world's best Parmesan, from the cows around Parma, Italy, is called "parmigiano-reggiano." It is semisweet and slightly salty, and it has a dry crumbly texture. It is also made from skim milk, which helps lower its fat content.

HOT PEPPER SAUCE: My favorite pepper sauce is an Asian one called Shriracha Chili Sauce and another from Jamaica called Jamaican Hell Fire. I'm also very fond of Pickapeppa sauce. They are found in the condiment aisle of the supermarket or a specialty store. If you don't find either, Tabasco will do fine.

PEPPERCORNS: Green peppercorns are harvested early and are best when pickled in brine. They have a salty taste like a caper, a bite like a pepper and a somewhat nutty texture. Black peppercorns are dried and are great when rough-ground at the last moment. White pepper is good used in light-colored sauces and mashed potatoes.

PENNE: A common pasta, penne is named because of its pointed ends, reminiscent of the pointed end of a fountain pen.

PIZZA CRUSTS: Make your own pizza dough from scratch, but when time is short, try pleasant Boboli, available in thin crust rounds. Prepared pizza dough can also be found in the dairy case.

PORCINI MUSHROOMS: These wild mushrooms are also known as cèpes. Dried porcini are used widely in Italian cooking; they contribute a rich, woodsy flavor to dishes. Packages of dried porcini may be found in the specialty section of most supermarkets and in Italian markets.

PHYLLO DOUGH: With the help of cooking spray, this makes a terrific pie crust. Find it in the freezer section of your supermarket. See techniques for using on pages 163 and 171.

RADICCHIO: This red-leaf Italian chicory with a deep purple-red hue and a somewhat hot taste is readily available and adds great flavor to salads. Peak season is midwinter to spring. It's terrific in salads as an alternative to tomatoes or as an enhancement.

ROASTED PEPPERS: The homemade version of these are the best, but the jarred variety are a convenient alternative. The peppers are bottled with water in 7½-ounce or larger jars and can usually be found alongside other Italian items in the supermarket.

SALSAS: These low-fat, flavorful toppings or dips can be purchased at the grocery store, either fresh at the deli area or jarred on the shelves. You can also make your own; it will stay fresh and high quality for four to five days. Try the recipes on pages 55 and 86.

STOCKS: These are flavor-packed liquids for almost all cooking in *Healthy Living*. They are readily available in the soup section of supermarkets, in low-sodium and low-fat versions.

You can also make your own more flavorful, less expensive stocks and store them in the freezer until ready to use. (Freeze stocks in ice cube trays till frozen, then empty these quarter-cup cubes into a freezer zip-top bag.)

Stock recipes are found on page 50.

the well-stocked kitchen

Trimming Fat From Stocks

For skimming fat from stocks (and soups or other liquids), trim a piece of wax paper the same size as the container the stock is in.

Gently lay wax paper directly on top of the stock, being careful not to let any liquid spill over it. Refrigerate to chill.

When ready, simply peel up the wax paper and all hardened fat will stick to it.

the well-stocked kitchen

TOMATO BASIL SAUCE: This all-round, perfect-for-many-uses sauce may be purchased jarred (on the grocer's shelves) or made fresh. If you opt to keep the purchased variety on hand, look for one such as Classico, made from naturally fresh ingredients with less than 2 grams of fat per serving. You may also want to try the recipe on page 59; it freezes beautifully in small freezer zip-top bags for up to three months.

WASHED SALAD PACKS AND FRESH VEGETABLES: Fresh Express and TKO market bags of washed, attractive, ready-to-eat salads come in 10- to 12-ounce bags. Some produce sections also offer cut vegetables—broccoli, cauliflower, carrots, celery—sold both separately and in combinations. They make for quick salads, stir-frying and fresh veggie platters.

WHOLE-WHEAT PASTRY FLOUR: Most easily found in natural food stores, this flour is the best choice for muffins, pancakes or waffles because it is finely milled from a soft wheat. It will make your whole-grain breads much lighter and less dense. Don't use for yeast breads, however, since this flour doesn't contain enough gluten for rising.

WINE: Wine is an excellent ingredient for adding flavor without caloric, fat or alcohol cost. Almost all of the alcohol evaporates during the cooking process. If you don't ordinarily have wine in your house when a recipe calls for it, buy wine splits (6.4 ounces or one-fourth of a standard wine bottle). Splits are easier to store and use up once opened.

WINE WITHOUT ALCOHOL: Because there are a number of people who choose not to use wine, even in cooking, you may want to substitute a good dealcoholized wine as an attractive ingredient.

These wines are distinguished by the fact that they are made from classic grapes, by classic methods and only subjected to the removal of the alcohol by a system of reverse osmosis. There are several producers; ask your supermarket for the best-selling brands and availability.

Some examples of dealcoholized wines are Sutter Home Fré and Ariel. Some grocery stores stock these in the juice aisle rather than with the traditional wines.

When cooking with these wines, it's best to split the amount, adding half at the beginning of the cooking process and half to freshen at the end.

VINEGARS: The zip and flavor that can be added to recipes through balsamic, raspberry, rice, red wine and tarragon vinegars can't be stressed enough. Plus, they add virtually no calories.

Balsamic is an incredibly complex vinegar that's great in salads and for marinades and finishing vegetables. Balsamic is aged in barrels of oak, chestnut, mulberry and juniper, picking up the flavors of each. Some are very old and expensive—but go for the mid-priced variety that doesn't rely on a fancy label for status selling.

Rice wine vinegar is a wonderful mild vinegar that is perfect for vinaigrettes and Asian salads. Chinese is mildest; Japanese does fine.

The Nutritional Top 10

Ever wish the science of nutrition could be pared down to a simple checklist? Good news! No longer must you stand dazed in the produce aisle, racking your brain for information about which fruits and veggies are rich in beta carotene (whatever that is).

Here's a shopping list to set you on a clear, no-brainer course: Simply toss these Top 10 foods into your grocery cart every week, make sure they get into your body, and you will have taken a giant step forward to good nutrition!

1. **BROCCOLI.** This is the best one-stop vegetable for beta carotene, fiber and vitamins C and A. It also contains sulforaphane, which blocks cancer growth.

2. **CHICKEN OR TURKEY.** These low-fat meats are great choices for building the body. Cook them in lean, flavorful ways.

3. **COLD-WATER SEAFOOD.** Buy salmon, tuna and swordfish. Valuable oils in fish provide protection against heart disease and other degenerative diseases such as arthritis. If you aren't a fish lover, become a ground flaxseed user; it's the only plant food that is rich in omega-3 fatty acids.

4. **LEGUMES.** These high-fiber beauties are also

high in protein and complex carbohydrates. Beans are loaded with phytochemicals and bioflavonoids that may help prevent cancer. They also lower LDL cholesterol levels in the blood, reducing heart disease risk. Soybeans are some of the best of this superfood group.

5. **ORANGES.** Fresh, whole citrus is a great source of vitamin C (oranges have the most). More than thirty studies have shown that vitamin C helps the body fight cancers. Oranges, along with mangoes, are also rich in bioflavonoids, which capture energy from the sun and become powerful boosters to our immune systems.

6. **SWEET POTATOES.** One of these (or two carrots) every other day provides enough beta carotene to protect against a host of diseases.

7. **SKIM OR LOW-FAT DAIRY PRODUCTS.** Milk, cheeses and yogurts are loaded with calcium and magnesium that keep blood pressure stable and bones strong. They're also excellent, low-fat sources of protein in convenient packaging.

8. **SPINACH.** This provides a bumper crop of vitamins A and C, and folic acid. It includes a bit of magnesium too, which helps control cancer, reduces the risk of stroke and heart disease, and may prevent osteoporosis.

9. **STRAWBERRIES AND TOMATOES.** These two foods are rich in substances that stimulate immune functions and slow degenerative diseases.

10. **WHOLE GRAINS.** Found in breads, cereals, crackers, rice and pasta, grains have fibers that lower cholesterol and blood pressure, and they may reduce the risk of colon cancer. Whole grains are loaded with B vitamins, calcium and magnesium, and vitamin E. These nutrients enhance the immune system and help prevent coronary artery disease. Oats are particularly valuable.

Don't forget two other little powerhouses: garlic and chili peppers. Garlic lowers cholesterol and blood pressure and boosts immunity. It also contains chemicals that may destroy cancer cells. Go for the real stuff, though. The capsules may not leave the garlic aroma with you, but they don't give you the health benefits either.

Chili peppers contain an antioxidant with many benefits. It boosts the immune system, protects against strokes and cancer-causing substances, lowers cholesterol and may even affect your mood by stimulating the release of endorphins!

Start with the freshest of ingredients and your end product will reflect the quality. Handpick what you eat and be selective.

the well-stocked kitchen

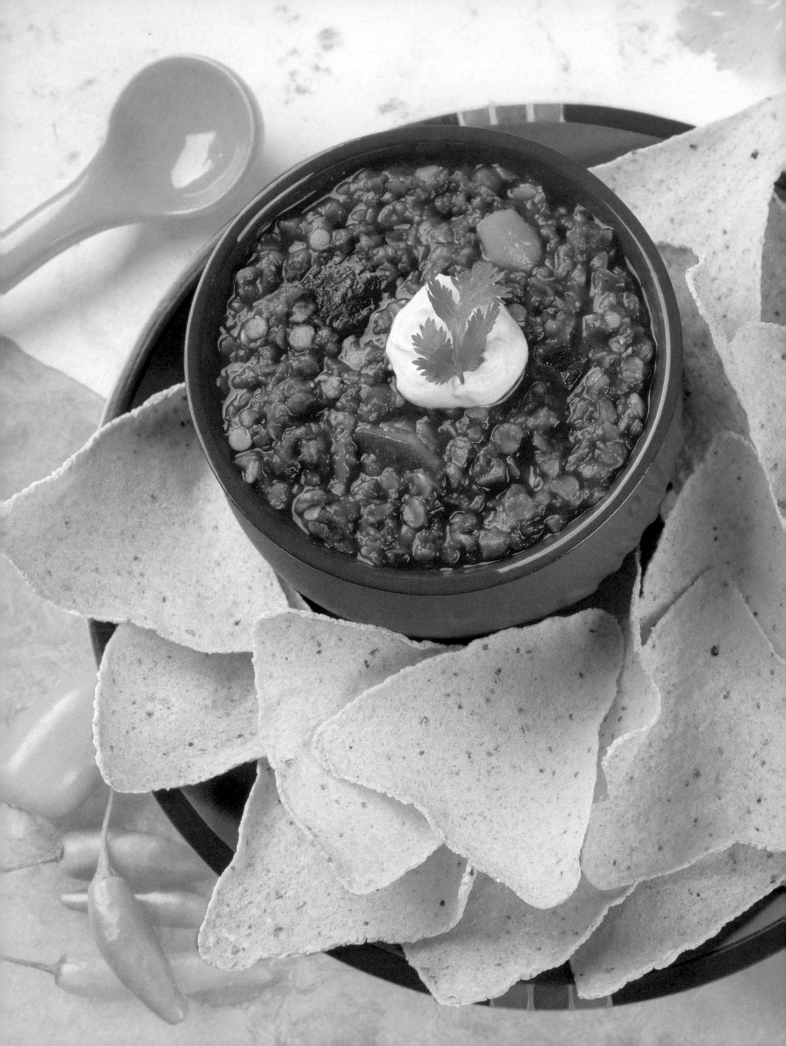

stocks, dressings, salsas and such

The secret of setting a "good table" is organization, which means planning ahead. Even if you have only half an hour to get a meal on the table, you can make it a healthy, balanced one, prepared from scratch, if you get—or even keep—most of the ingredients ready ahead of time.

On the following pages you will find a grouping of stock recipes—dressings, spreads, sauces, salsas and such. Although most are used in recipes within *Healthy Living,* you can mix and match them, creating your own special dish. Here is the beauty of this kind of fresh and flavorful cuisine: If you start with good ingredients and a little guidance, you can make up your own rules.

Always have stocks on hand for steaming vegetables, cooking pasta and rice, and making soups and sauces. They provide flavor in a light way.

Cook stocks in large quantities and chill to allow all the fat to rise to the surface. A new easy way to skim the fat is with a piece of wax paper trimmed to the size of the container holding the stock. Gently lay it on top of the stock and skim off the fat, then freeze or refrigerate stock.

Pictured: Red lentil chili made with chicken stock
(pg. 103)

Homemade Stocks

Hearty Meat Stock

3 to 4 pounds chicken pieces (or beef or veal bones with meat on them)
6 black peppercorns
2 carrots, sliced
2 cloves garlic, minced
1 medium onion, chopped
1 stalk celery with leaves, sliced
1 bay leaf
2 Tbsp. chopped fresh parsley (or 1 Tbsp. dried)
1 tsp. salt

Cover chicken with water; add peppercorns. Simmer uncovered for 30 minutes. Add remaining ingredients. Cover and simmer for 2 additional hours (4 additional hours for beef or veal). Strain stock and remove chicken. Use deboned chicken in salads or recipes calling for cubed chicken.

Chill stock until the fat can be skimmed off easily. The stock is then ready to use, or it can be frozen for use later.

1 serving = 4 oz. or ½ cup.

Per Serving: 10 Calories

Protein 1.8 gr.	Carb. less than 1 gr.
Fat less than 1 gr.	Cal. from fat 0%
Chol. 0 mg.	Sodium 120 mg.

Trimmings Stock

scrubbed vegetable tops, peelings and scraps
salt (or low-sodium soy sauce)
onions (or garlic) for flavoring as desired
herbs as desired (choose from bay leaves, rosemary, basil and others)

Load a heavy pot with scrubbed vegetable scraps. (These can be collected for up to a week and stored in the refrigerator in a plastic bag.) Cover the scraps with water; add a pinch of salt. Salt is optional, but it will draw nutrients into the stock. Add onions and your favorite herbs. Cover the pot and let simmer for 1 to 2 hours, stirring occasionally.

Let cool; strain and refrigerate or freeze. Stock will keep for 8 to 10 days in the refrigerator. Freeze the stock in either pint-sized containers or ice cube trays (store frozen cubes in plastic bags). One cube equals ¼ cup stock.

1 serving = 4 oz. or ½ cup.

Per Serving: 4 Calories

Protein 0 gr.	Carb. less than 1 gr.
Fat 0 gr.	Cal. from fat 0%
Chol. 0 mg.	Sodium 120 mg.

Tips for Making Stocks

Cook stocks in large quantities and chill to allow all the fat to rise to the surface. Skim off this fat, then freeze or refrigerate stock.

Salad Dressings

Honey-Orange Vinaigrette

½ cup orange juice
1 Tbsp. honey
½ cup balsamic vinegar
½ tsp. creole seasoning
1 tsp. Pickapeppa sauce (or hot pepper sauce)
juice of ½ lemon
1 Tbsp. chopped fresh herbs (cilantro, basil, rosemary, thyme)

Mix together all ingredients. Refrigerate.
Makes 10 servings, 2 Tbsp. each.

Per Serving: 12 Calories

Protein 0 gr.	Carb. 3 gr.
Fat 0 gr.	Cal. from fat 0%
Chol. 0 mg.	Sodium 53 mg.

Greek Vinaigrette

¼ cup olive oil
1¼ cups rice wine vinegar
¾ cup chicken stock (fat-free/low salt)
¼ cup Dijon mustard
½ cup pepperoncini juice
1 Tbsp. minced garlic
1 Tbsp. minced shallots
1 tsp. creole seasoning
2 Tbsp. chopped fresh herbs (cilantro, basil, rosemary, thyme)
1 Tbsp. chopped fresh oregano (or 1 tsp. dried)

In a large bowl, whisk together all ingredients. Refrigerate.
Makes 25 servings, 2 Tbsp. each.

Per Serving: 21 Calories

Protein 0 gr.	Carb. 1 gr.
Fat 2 gr.	Cal. from fat 66%
Chol. 0 mg.	Sodium 139 mg.

Herbal Vinaigrette

2 cups chicken stock (fat-free/low salt)
¼ cup olive oil
1 cup balsamic vinegar
1 tsp. cornstarch
1 Tbsp. cold water
2 tsp. minced garlic
¼ tsp. cracked black pepper
1 tsp. creole seasoning
1 Tbsp. chopped fresh thyme
1 Tbsp. chopped fresh parsley
1 Tbsp. chopped fresh basil
1 Tbsp. chopped fresh oregano
1 Tbsp. chopped fresh chives

Heat together chicken stock, olive oil and vinegar.

In a separate bowl, whisk cornstarch together with cold water. Add to stock mixture and let simmer for 1 minute to thicken.

Take off heat and cool. Add remaining ingredients and refrigerate.

Makes 25 servings, 2 Tbsp. each.

Per Serving: 21 Calories

Protein 0 gr.	Carb. 1 gr.
Fat 2 gr.	Cal. from fat 66%
Chol. 0 mg.	Sodium 145 mg.

Homemade Dressings Are Easy and Not Fattening!

It's easy to pick up a bottle of fat-free dressing at the store, but with scarcely more effort, you can whip up delicious homemade versions of your store-bought favorites.

Don't despair that these dressings seem to have such a high percentage of calories from fat— the calories are so low that even a gram of fat looks like a lot. When used in a recipe, the percentage normalizes.

These salad dressings rely on the mild flavors of wonderful vinegars, herbs, spices and chicken stock. I often use skim-milk cheeses to thicken these dressings, so precious little oil is added.

Salad Dressings (continued)

Citrus Vinaigrette

2 Tbsp. olive oil
2/3 cup rice wine vinegar
1/3 cup orange juice
1 Tbsp. Dijon mustard
1 tsp. honey
2 tsp. minced garlic
1 Tbsp. minced shallots
1/2 tsp. creole seasoning
2 Tbsp. chopped fresh cilantro

Mix all ingredients together. Refrigerate.
Makes 12 servings, 2 Tbsp. each.

Per Serving: 30 Calories

Protein 0 gr.	Carb. 3 gr.
Fat 2 gr.	Cal. from fat 62%
Chol. 0 mg.	Sodium 62 mg.

Green Goddess Dressing

1 cup nonfat cottage cheese
1/2 cup cider vinegar
2 stalks celery, diced
1/2 cup spinach leaves, washed and stemmed
1/3 cup fresh parsley
1/2 tsp. cracked black pepper
2 Tbsp. chopped fresh tarragon
1 Tbsp. lemon juice
2 scallions, sliced thin
1 tsp. Mrs. Dash seasoning
1/2 tsp. creole seasoning

Blend cottage cheese in blender or food processor until smooth. Add remaining ingredients and blend well. Refrigerate.
Makes 12 servings, 2 Tbsp. each.

Per Serving: 14 Calories

Protein 2 gr.	Carb. 1.5 gr.
Fat 0 gr.	Cal. from fat 0%
Chol. 1 mg.	Sodium 54 mg.

Cucumber Dill Dressing

6 oz. light cream cheese
1/3 cup farmer's cheese
1 cup skim milk
1 cup cucumbers, peeled, seeded and chopped
1 1/2 Tbsp. Dijon mustard
2 cloves garlic, minced
1/4 tsp. cracked black pepper
1 tsp. creole seasoning
1 Tbsp. olive oil
juice of 1 lemon
1/2 tsp. Tabasco
2 Tbsp. chopped fresh dill

Blend cheeses and skim milk in a blender. Add all other ingredients except dill and blend until smooth. Stir in dill.
Makes 24 servings, 4 Tbsp. each.

Per Serving: 38 Calories

Protein 1.5 gr.	Carb. 1 gr.
Fat 3 gr.	Cal. from fat 71%
Chol. 3 mg.	Sodium 34 mg.

Make Your Own Flavored Vinegar

You can make your own flavored vinegars easily and inexpensively.

To Make Herb Vinegar:

Start with a wine vinegar, cider vinegar or rice wine vinegar base, then add fresh herbs of your choosing, such as tarragon or basil. Whole garlic cloves may be added as well.

To Make Fruit-Flavored Vinegar:

Add top-quality berries such as raspberries to a wine vinegar, cider vinegar or rice wine vinegar base. Use 2 cups fruit for every 2 cups of vinegar. Let the mixture steep, covered, in a wide-mouthed jar for a week, then transfer all to a clean bottle and refrigerate. May use for 6 weeks.

Salad Dressings (continued)

Horseradish Dressing

3 Tbsp. grated fresh horseradish
16 oz. nonfat plain yogurt
2 Tbsp. minced shallots
¼ tsp. white pepper
½ tsp. creole seasoning
1 tsp. Mrs. Dash seasoning
1 Tbsp. low-sodium soy sauce
2 Tbsp. rice wine vinegar
juice of 2 lemons
⅓ cup orange juice concentrate

Use fresh horseradish, if possible. Peel and grate very fine.

Whisk horseradish together with remaining ingredients. Chill.

Makes 25 servings, 2 Tbsp. each.

Per Serving: 14 Calories

Protein 1 gr.	Carb. 2.5 gr.
Fat 0 gr.	Cal. from fat 0%
Chol. 0 mg.	Sodium 98 mg.

Peppercorn-Parmesan Dressing

1 cup nonfat buttermilk
¼ cup grated Parmesan cheese
⅓ cup nonfat sour cream
¼ cup light mayonnaise
2 Tbsp. lemon juice
2 tsp. cracked black pepper
¼ tsp. salt

Combine all ingredients in a bowl; stir well with wire whisk. Cover and chill. Perfect served over mixed greens.

Makes 12 servings, 2 Tbsp. each.

Per Serving: 33 Calories

Protein 1 gr.	Carb. 1 gr.
Fat 2 gr.	Cal. from fat 53%
Chol. 2 mg.	Sodium 100 mg.

Caesar Salad Dressing

2 tsp. spicy hot mustard
1 tsp. anchovy paste
1 clove garlic, minced
½ cup nonfat buttermilk
¼ cup grated Parmesan cheese
2 Tbsp. white wine*
2 Tbsp. red wine vinegar
½ tsp. creole seasoning
1 Tbsp. chopped fresh parsley
1 Tbsp. lemon juice
1 Tbsp. olive oil

* or substitute dealcoholized wine or chicken stock (fat-free/low salt)

Combine mustard, anchovy paste and garlic in a small bowl; stir well. Add remaining ingredients, stirring with a wire whisk until blended. Cover and chill. Try this over mixed greens.

Makes 8 servings, 2 Tbsp. each.

Per Serving: 39 Calories

Protein 2 gr.	Carb. 1.5 gr.
Fat 2.5 gr.	Cal. from fat 58%
Chol. 2.5 mg.	Sodium 152 mg.

stocks, dressings, salsas and such

Storing Horseradish

Fresh horseradish is found in your supermarket's produce section and can be stored in airtight plastic bags for up to 3 weeks. Peel and cut out the fibrous core just before grating.

Bottled horseradish can be found in the refrigerated case of the supermarket. Once opened, it loses its flavor within 4 weeks. You can freeze it for longer use by spooning tablespoons onto a baking sheet and freezing till solid. Then transfer them to an airtight plastic bag for use over the next 6 months.

Salad Dressings (continued)

Roasted Garlic Dijon Vinaigrette

5 full heads garlic, roasted* and puréed
1 tsp. creole seasoning
½ cup rice wine vinegar
2 Tbsp. honey
½ cup Dijon mustard
1 tsp. cracked black pepper
1 tsp. Mrs. Dash Garlic and Herb Seasoning
1 cup chicken stock (fat-free/low salt)
¼ cup olive oil

* To roast garlic, chop stems off garlic heads until the flesh of the cloves is visible. Place open ends down on very lightly oiled baking pan. Cover with aluminum foil and bake in 350-degree oven until soft, about 45 minutes to 1 hour. Remove from oven and allow to cool. Then squeeze out all the tender and flavorful flesh from the heads. Discard emptied heads.

Combine all ingredients except oil in food processor or blender. Blend together. While blending, slowly add oil and continue processing until oil is incorporated and dressing is well blended. Refrigerate.
Makes 25 servings, 2 Tbsp. each.

Per Serving: 36 Calories

Protein 1 gr.   Carb. 3.5 gr.
Fat 2 gr.   Cal. from fat 58%
Chol. 0 mg.   Sodium 110 mg.

Extra-Smooth Vinaigrette

For an extra-smooth vinaigrette, combine the ingredients and an ice cube in a screw-top jar and shake vigorously. Discard the ice cube once the dressing is mixed.

Dressing in a Hurry

½ cup balsamic or rice wine vinegar
⅓ cup chicken stock (fat-free/low salt)
1 pkg. dried Italian dressing mix
1 Tbsp. olive oil

Pour vinegar and chicken stock into shakable container with lid. Add dressing mix and olive oil. Shake well and refrigerate.
Makes 8 servings, 2 Tbsp. each.

Per Serving: 15 Calories

Protein 0 gr.   Carb. 1 gr.
Fat 1.2 gr.   Cal. from fat 79%
Chol. 0 mg.   Sodium 320 mg.

Cumin-Dijon Dressing

3 Tbsp. lemon juice
1 Tbsp. olive oil
1 Tbsp. red wine vinegar
2 Tbsp. chicken stock (fat-free/low salt)
1 tsp. cumin
1 tsp. Dijon mustard
2 cloves garlic, minced
½ tsp. creole seasoning

Whisk ingredients together. This dressing can be used with salads and is a delicious addition to pita sandwiches.
Makes 4 servings, 2 Tbsp. each.

Per Serving: 31 Calories

Protein 0 gr.   Carb. 0 gr.
Fat 3.4 gr.   Cal. from fat 98%
Chol. 0 mg.   Sodium 150 mg.

Special Salsas

Pineapple Tomato Salsa

1 pineapple, diced
1 red bell pepper, cut into strips
2 plum tomatoes, diced
juice of 1 lime
1 Tbsp. chopped fresh cilantro
1/4 tsp. dried coriander seed
1 tsp. creole seasoning

Mix all ingredients. Refrigerate at least 1 hour to blend flavors. This salsa will keep in the refrigerator for 4 to 5 days. Serve with sandwiches or salads.

Makes 4 servings, 1/3 cup each.

Per Serving: 32 Calories

Protein 0 gr.
Fat 0 gr.
Chol. 0 mg.

Carb. 8 gr.
Cal. from fat 0%
Sodium 268 mg.

Tropical Salsa

1 papaya, diced
1 ripe mango, diced
1/2 pineapple, diced
1 red bell pepper, cut into strips
1 tomato, diced
juice of 1 lemon
juice of 1 lime
1 Tbsp. chopped fresh cilantro
1 Tbsp. coconut rum (or 1 tsp. coconut extract)
1/4 tsp. dried coriander seed
1 tsp. creole seasoning

Mix all ingredients. Refrigerate to blend flavors. Serve as a sensational side for sandwiches or as a bed for grilled fish, poultry or beef.

Makes 8 servings, 1/3 cup each.

Per Serving: 40 Calories

Protein 0 gr.
Fat 0 gr.
Chol. 0 mg.

Carb. 10 gr.
Cal. from fat 0%
Sodium 136 mg.

Black Bean and Corn Salsa

2 cups black beans, drained and rinsed
1 cup frozen corn kernels, thawed
2 plum tomatoes, diced
1/2 red onion, minced
1 serrano pepper, minced
1 Tbsp. chopped fresh cilantro
1 Tbsp. olive oil
4 cloves garlic, minced
juice of 2 limes
1 Tbsp. balsamic vinegar
1 tsp. cumin
2 tsp. hot pepper sauce
1 tsp. creole seasoning

In a large bowl, combine all ingredients and mix well. Allow to marinate at least 1 hour before serving.

Makes 10 servings, 1/3 cup each.

Per Serving: 79 Calories

Protein 4 gr.
Fat 1.5 gr.
Chol. 0 mg.

Carb. 13 gr.
Cal. from fat 17%
Sodium 118 mg.

Lemon Lovers

Choose lemons and limes with smooth, brightly colored skin— they should be firm, plump and heavy for their size. One medium lemon yields 3 Tbsp. juice (and 2 to 3 tsp. zest).

Buy lemons in peak season. Squeeze the juice and freeze it in ice cube trays. Once solid, turn them into heavy- weight plastic bags, seal tightly and freeze for up to 6 months.

Lemons at room tem- perature will yield more juice than refrigerated ones. Popping them into the microwave for 30 seconds on high will also release more juice. Cut them lengthwise for the best squeezing.

BBQ Sauces & Marinades

Balsamic Marinade

3 cups chicken stock (fat-free/low salt)
½ cup olive oil
2 cups balsamic vinegar
1 Tbsp. cornstarch
2 Tbsp. water
1 Tbsp. minced garlic
1 tsp. cracked black pepper
1 Tbsp. chopped fresh thyme
2 Tbsp. chopped fresh cilantro
1 Tbsp. chopped fresh basil
½ Tbsp. chopped fresh oregano
½ Tbsp. chopped chives
1 Tbsp. Pickapeppa sauce (or hot pepper sauce)
¼ cup orange juice
juice of 1 lime
1 serrano or jalapeño pepper, seeded and diced
2 tsp. creole seasoning

Heat chicken stock, oil and vinegar. In a separate bowl, blend together the cornstarch and water. Add to the stock mixture. Gently boil for 1 minute to thicken.

Remove from heat and cool. Add remaining ingredients and refrigerate.

Use for marinating meats and vegetables. Marinating time can vary from 15 minutes to overnight.

Makes 50 servings, 2 Tbsp. each.

Per Serving: 21 Calories

Protein 0 gr.   Carb. 1 gr.
Fat 2 gr.   Cal. from fat 85%
Chol. 0 mg.   Sodium 43 mg.

Citrus BBQ Sauce

2 cups KC Masterpiece BBQ Sauce (or your favorite BBQ sauce)
1 can (6 oz.) orange juice concentrate
1 tsp. creole seasoning
1 Tbsp. Jamaican jerk seasoning
juice of ½ lime

In a medium bowl, whisk together all ingredients. Refrigerate. Excellent on chicken, pork chops and turkey cutlets.

Makes 3 cups, 24 servings, 2 Tbsp. per serving.

Per Serving: 29 Calories

Protein 0 gr.   Carb. 6 gr.
Fat less than 1 gr.   Cal. from fat 0%
Chol. 0 mg.   Sodium 205 mg.

European Marinade

½ cup lime or lemon juice
2 tsp. dried thyme
2 cloves garlic, minced
1 Tbsp. olive oil
½ tsp. salt
½ tsp. cracked black pepper

Combine all ingredients. Use to marinate skinned chicken, meat, fish or seafood for 3 to 4 hours or overnight.

Makes ½ cup, 4 servings, 2 Tbsp. per serving.

Per Serving: 26 Calories

Protein 0 gr.   Carb. 2 gr.
Fat 2 gr.   Cal. from fat 69%
Chol. 0 mg.   Sodium 267 mg.

Marinate It!

Marinades flavor and tenderize foods. Most marinades contain an acid ingredient (like lemon or lime juice, vinegar or wine) that tenderizes tough cuts of meat.

Always marinate food in a glass or plastic container, never metal. Allow the marinade to cover the food. Food can also be marinated in a large zip-top plastic bag. Turn the bag occasionally to distribute the marinade.

Unused marinade may be refrigerated for up to 2 weeks.

Used marinade must be frozen, then thawed for future use. Boil before using.

BBQ Sauces & Marinades (continued)

Jamaican Marinade

¼ cup olive oil
2 Tbsp. Jamaican jerk seasoning
¼ cup orange juice
2 Tbsp. low-sodium soy sauce
¼ cup white vinegar
1 Tbsp. dark Jamaican rum (optional)
juice of 1 lime
1 Scotch bonnet or habanero pepper,
   seeded and minced
2 cloves garlic, minced
½ cup chopped white onions
2 green onions, chopped
½ tsp. creole seasoning

Slowly add the olive oil to the jerk seasoning, stirring with a wire whisk. Then add all remaining ingredients; stir. Refrigerate. Use to marinate chicken, pork and lean beef.

Makes 1½ cups of marinade, about 12 servings, 2 Tbsp. per serving.

Per Serving: 47 Calories

Protein 0 gr.   Carb. 1.5 gr.
Fat 4 gr.   Cal. from fat 83%
Chol. 0 mg.   Sodium 131 mg.

Tropical Marinade

⅓ cup unsweetened pineapple juice
⅓ cup low-sodium soy sauce
⅓ cup sherry or chicken stock
   (fat-free/low salt)
2 cloves garlic, minced
2 Tbsp. chopped fresh parsley
   (or 1 Tbsp. dried)
½ tsp. cracked black pepper

Combine all ingredients. Use to marinate skinned chicken, beef, fish or seafood for 3 to 4 hours or overnight. (The marinade adds no significant calories to the meat.)

Makes 1 cup, 8 servings, 2 Tbsp. per serving.

Per Serving: 9 Calories

Protein 0 gr.   Carb. 2 gr.
Fat 0 gr.   Cal. from fat 0%
Chol. 0 mg.   Sodium 387 mg.

Oriental Sauce

¼ cup chicken stock (fat-free/low salt)
2 Tbsp. dry sherry or dealcoholized
   wine
2 Tbsp. hoisin sauce
2 Tbsp. low-sodium soy sauce
1½ tsp. minced ginger root
2 cloves garlic, minced
1 tsp. Shriracha Chili Sauce (or hot
   pepper sauce)

Mix together all ingredients and refrigerate. Use as either a marinade or BBQ sauce.

Makes ¾ cup, 6 servings, 2 Tbsp. per serving.

Per Serving: 26 Calories

Protein 0 gr.   Carb. 6 gr.
Fat 0 gr.   Cal. from fat 0
Chol. 0 mg.   Sodium 515 mg.

stocks, dressings, salsas and such

Pointers About Peppers

The undisputed hottest peppers in the world are those flaming orange gems known as Scotch bonnets from Jamaica and habaneros from Mexico.

They are so similar that some say they're one and the same (but Jamaicans disagree).

Whichever you choose, a little goes a long way. Wear rubber gloves, and be careful not to get the oil on your skin or in your eyes. Removing the seeds and membranes will moderate the heat.

If you can't find the real thing, you can substitute fresh serrano peppers or dried habaneros.

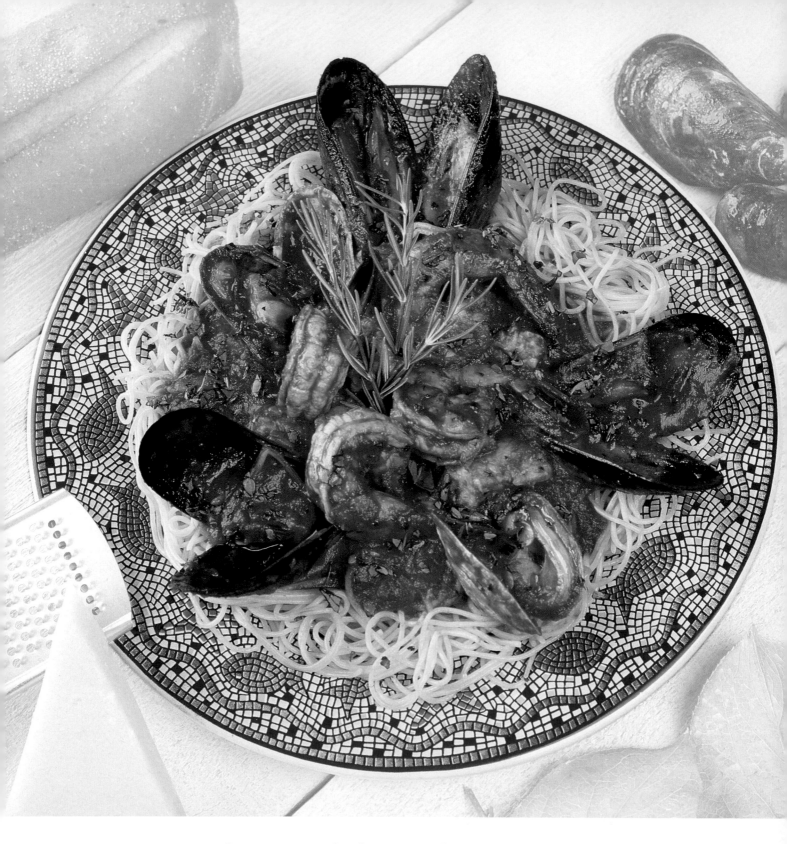

Mediterranean Seafood Stew—made from Tomato Basil Sauce
This delicious, all-round, perfect-for-many-uses sauce is a wonderful accompaniment for many recipes—and it may be made in large quantities and frozen in zip-top bags for later use.

Sauces

Tomato Basil Sauce

1 Tbsp. olive oil
2 white onions, diced medium
2 tsp. minced garlic
½ cup minced shallots
1 Tbsp. chopped fresh thyme
1 tsp. chopped fresh rosemary
1 Tbsp. chopped fresh oregano
2 Tbsp. chopped fresh basil
5 tomatoes, skinned, seeded and diced*
1 can (32 oz.) whole tomatoes
1 Tbsp. creole seasoning
1 Tbsp. Mrs. Dash Garlic and Herb
   Seasoning

* Tomatoes are easily skinned by immersing
  them in boiling water for 10 seconds.
  Remove with slotted spoon. Skins will
  "slip off."

Sauté onions, garlic, shallots and herbs in olive oil until onions are transparent, about 3 to 4 minutes.

Add fresh and canned tomatoes. Cook for 5 minutes at full heat. Lower heat and continue cooking until sauce has reduced by one-third.

Add seasonings. Cook for about 1½ hours, stirring occasionally. Leave chunky; do not grind or blend.

This sauce may be made in large quantities and frozen (after cooling) in zip-top bags for later use. Microwave or place in refrigerator to thaw.

Makes 14 servings, ½ cup each.

Per Serving: 40 Calories

Protein 1 gr.	Carb. 7 gr.
Fat 1 gr.	Cal. from fat 25%
Chol. 0 mg.	Sodium 240 mg.

Fire-Roasted Pepper Sauce

1 tsp. olive oil
½ red onion, diced
2 cloves garlic, minced
8 red bell peppers, fire-roasted*
8 pablano peppers, fire-roasted*
2 Tbsp. Lea and Perrins
   Worcestershire for Chicken
2 cups chicken stock (fat-free/low salt)
1 Tbsp. creole seasoning

* To fire-roast peppers, slice peppers in half
  lengthwise, core and remove the seeds.
  Put the sliced peppers directly on the rack
  of a preheated broiler, cut side down. Broil
  for about 5 minutes, until the skin blisters.
  Transfer the roasted peppers to a tightly
  sealed plastic bag. Close it and leave
  them for 10 to 15 minutes. When cool,
  the charred skin can be rubbed easily
  from the peppers and discarded.

Heat olive oil in saucepan. Add onion and garlic, and begin to sauté. Add peppers, Lea and Perrins Worcestershire for Chicken, chicken stock and seasoning. Cook until the sauce begins to reduce.

Perfect as a sauce for grilled fish, poultry or beef, or as a dipping sauce for sandwiches.

Makes 25 servings, ¼ cup each.

Per Serving: 16 Calories

Protein 0 gr.	Carb. 3 gr.
Fat less than 1 gr.	Cal. from fat 15%
Chol. 0 mg.	Sodium 142 mg.

stocks, dressings, salsas and such

Pleasing Veggie Purées

Vegetable purées added to sauces and side dishes can be a clever way of coaxing finicky eaters to try a dreaded vegetable. Cook them, throw them in a blender, add some chicken stock and purée. You've just made a sauce for grilled meat. Try laying the meat on the sauce instead of putting the sauce on the meat.

Purées take well to advance preparation and gentle reheating over a double boiler or in a microwave. Keep them tightly wrapped in the refrigerator so they don't dry out.

Sensational Spreads

Spicy Dijonnaise

1 cup light mayonnaise
½ cup nonfat plain yogurt
1½ tsp. Pickapeppa sauce (or hot pepper sauce)
1½ tsp. Sriracha chili sauce (or Tabasco sauce)
¼ cup Dijon mustard
½ tsp. curry powder
½ tsp. creole seasoning
3 green onions, diced
1 Tbsp. chopped fresh cilantro
2 cloves garlic, minced
½ tsp. black pepper

Mix together mayonnaise, yogurt, sauces, mustard, curry and seasoning. Add onions, cilantro, garlic and pepper. Serve as a flavorful spread for sandwiches.
Makes 30 servings, 1 Tbsp. each.

Per Serving: 24 Calories

Protein 0 gr.	Carb. 1 gr.
Fat 2 gr.	Cal. from fat 78%
Chol. 3 mg.	Sodium 49 mg.

Garlic Aioli

1 cup light mayonnaise
½ cup nonfat plain yogurt
½ tsp. creole seasoning
1 Tbsp. minced shallots
2 tsp. chopped fresh herbs (cilantro, basil, rosemary, thyme)
4 cloves garlic, minced
juice of ½ lemon

Mix together all ingredients. Great on turkey burgers, fish sandwiches or any special sandwich.
Makes 25 servings, 1 Tbsp. each.

Per Serving: 28 Calories

Protein 0 gr.	Carb. 1 gr.
Fat 2.5 gr.	Cal. from fat 80%
Chol. 3 mg.	Sodium 25 mg.

Bean and Garlic Pesto

1½ Tbsp. olive oil, divided
3 cloves garlic, left whole
2 cups white cannelini beans, rinsed and drained
¼ cup lemon juice
2 Tbsp. chicken stock (fat-free/low salt)
1 Tbsp. chopped fresh parsley
1 tsp. hot pepper sauce
¼ tsp. creole seasoning
1 tsp. chopped fresh rosemary
3 Tbsp. roasted red pepper, finely chopped (purchased)

In an ovenproof skillet over medium-high heat, warm ½ Tbsp. of the olive oil. Add garlic and sauté until lightly browned, 3 to 5 minutes. Leave garlic in skillet and bake in oven at 400 degrees until well-browned and softened, 15 to 20 minutes.

In a food processor or blender, purée the rest of the ingredients with roasted garlic and remaining 1 Tbsp. of oil.

This goes perfectly with vegetable baguettes, pocket pitas or any sensational sandwich. Also excellent with whole-grain crackers as a protein snack.
Makes 10 servings, ¼ cup each.

Per Serving: 68 Calories

Protein 3 gr.	Carb. 10 gr.
Fat 2 gr.	Cal. from fat 28%
Chol. 0 mg.	Sodium 54 mg.

Mayo Mania

When it comes to mayo, don't get caught in the fat-free trap. If a product says "fat-free," you must ask, "Then what is in it?" The best choice for mayonnaise is the reduced-fat or light variety; it is low in fat only because it's been whipped with added air and water. The fat-free choice is loaded with multiple sugars, chemicals and food dyes.

You can avoid a lot of mayo by focusing on Dijon mustard, salsa or aioli-type spread made with nonfat yogurt.

Crowd-Pleaser Dips for Chips

Black Bean Dip

2 cans (15 oz. each) black beans,
    drained and rinsed
4 Tbsp. finely chopped canned or
    fresh jalapeño peppers
2 Tbsp. red wine vinegar
2 tsp. chili powder (or to taste)
½ tsp. creole seasoning
¼ tsp. cumin
1 Tbsp. minced onion
1 tsp. minced garlic
1 Tbsp. chopped fresh parsley

Place in blender the beans, peppers, vinegar, chili powder, seasoning and cumin. Blend until smooth. Transfer the mixture to a bowl.
   Stir in the onion, garlic and parsley.
   Makes 12 servings, ⅓ cup each.

Per Serving: 117 Calories

Protein 8 gr.	Carb. 21 gr.
Fat 0 gr.	Cal. from fat 0%
Chol. 0 mg.	Sodium 68 mg.

Salmon Dip

5 oz. smoked salmon fillet
1 tsp. low-sodium soy sauce
juice of ½ lemon
1 tsp. lime juice
1 Tbsp. chopped fresh parsley (or
    1 tsp. dried)
1 tsp. Worcestershire sauce
½ tsp. grated fresh wasabi or
    horseradish
1 tsp. minced ginger root
dash of Tabasco sauce
dash of cracked black pepper

Roughly chop salmon. Mix it with all ingredients. Very good with whole-wheat toast points.
   Makes 4 servings, ¼ cup each.

Per Serving: 49 Calories

Protein 8 gr.	Carb. 3 gr.
Fat less than 1 gr.	Cal. from fat 6%
Chol. 16 mg.	Sodium 97 mg.

Creamy Herb Dip

4 oz. light cream cheese, softened
¼ cup nonfat sour cream
3 Tbsp. chopped fresh chives or
    scallions
1 Tbsp. chopped fresh dill
½ tsp. creole seasoning
1 tsp. Mrs. Dash seasoning
1 tsp. prepared horseradish

Stir cream cheese into sour cream until smooth. Mix in chives, dill, seasonings and horseradish. Spoon into a small bowl. Wonderful with fresh vegetables.
   Makes 4 servings, ¼ cup each.

Per Serving: 24 Calories

Protein 4 gr.	Carb. 1.5 gr.
Fat 0 gr.	Cal. from fat 0%
Chol. 1 mg.	Sodium 147 mg.

stocks, dressings, salsas and such

Baked Tortilla Chips

Be sure to try the new baked tortilla chips—a tasty, crunchy alternative to the high-fat, fried versions. Generally, 25 chips or so give less than 1 gram of fat. They serve as great dippers for fat-free bean dips and salsas and are a way to add texture to salads.

You can also make your own baked chips. Lightly spray tortillas with cooking spray and season lightly to taste with salt, pepper and/or chili powder. Cut into 12 wedges and bake at 350 degrees until crisp.

stocks, dressings, salsas and such

Tropical Fruit Tips

Choose mangoes and papayas with unblem-ished, yellow skin blushed with red. The larger the fruit, the higher the fruit-to-seed ratio. Ripe mangoes will yield to gentle pressure and have a tropical fra-grance. Avoid those with shriveled or black-speckled skin.

Refrigerate ripe fruit in a plastic bag for up to 5 days. Place underripe fruit in a paper bag (pierce bag with tip of knife) with a banana at room temperature for 1 to 3 days. Green, rock-hard mangoes and papayas will probably never ripen.

Refreshing Relishes

White Bean Relish

3 cups cooked white beans, drained
juice of 1 lime
¾ cup Herbal Vinaigrette (pg. 51)
1 tsp. creole seasoning
2 tsp. minced garlic
2 Tbsp. minced shallots
4 Tbsp. chopped fresh cilantro
3 Tbsp. each diced yellow, red and
    green bell peppers
1 plum tomato, seeded and diced

Mix all ingredients together with beans. Refrigerate.
Use as a sensational side for salads, sand-wiches and grilled vegetables.
Makes 10 servings, ⅓ cup each.

Per Serving: 85 Calories

Protein 5 gr.	Carb. 14 gr.
Fat 1 gr.	Cal. from fat 17%
Chol. 0 mg.	Sodium 108 mg.

Mango Chutney

½ ripe mango, cut in strips
1 Tbsp. hot mango chutney
½ red bell pepper, cut into strips
¼ cup orange juice
juice of ½ lime
1 Tbsp. fresh coriander or cilantro
½ tsp. creole seasoning
1 Tbsp. low-sodium soy sauce

Mix all ingredients. Refrigerate to blend flavors.
Makes 6 servings, ¼ cup each.

Per Serving: 25 Calories

Protein 0 gr.	Carb. 6 gr.
Fat 0 gr.	Cal. from fat 0%
Chol. 0 mg.	Sodium 184 mg.

Papaya Ginger Relish

1 papaya, diced
1 Tbsp. ginger root, cut into fine strips
1 red bell pepper, cut into strips
1 serrano or Hungarian pepper, diced
juice of 1 lemon
½ cup orange juice
2 chives, cut in 1-inch lengths
1 tsp. creole seasoning

Mix all ingredients. Refrigerate to blend fla-vors. Super with grilled fish, seafood or chicken, or as a side dish for a sandwich.
Makes 6 servings, ⅓ cup each.

Per Serving: 32 Calories

Protein 0 gr.	Carb. 8 gr.
Fat 0 gr.	Cal. from fat 0%
Chol. 0 mg.	Sodium 180 mg.

Fruit Toppings

Apple Compote

¾ cup water
¼ cup honey
2 Granny Smith apples, peeled, cored
  and sliced
1 tsp. cornstarch
⅛ tsp. nutmeg
¼ tsp. cinnamon

Combine water and honey in saucepan; add apples. Bring to boil, then reduce heat and simmer until apples are tender. Remove apples from liquid.

Dissolve cornstarch in a portion of the liquid. Bring remaining liquid back to a boil and add cornstarch mixture. Cook another minute to thicken, then remove from heat. Add spices and stir. Gently fold in apples. Great over pancakes or frozen yogurt.

Makes 8 servings, ¼ cup each.

Per Serving: 53 Calories

Protein 0 gr.	Carb. 14 gr.
Fat 0 gr.	Cal. from fat 0%
Chol. 0 mg.	Sodium 1 mg.

Yogurt Fruit Sauce

4 cups nonfat plain yogurt
1 cup orange juice
½ cup honey
2 Tbsp. grated orange rind
2 Tbsp. grated lemon rind
½ Tbsp. nutmeg
fresh fruit, chopped

Whisk together yogurt, orange juice, honey, orange rind, lemon rind and nutmeg. Chill.

When serving, mix in 2 Tbsp. chopped fresh fruit per ¼ cup serving of yogurt sauce. Wonderful with pancakes, waffles or French toast, or use as a dipping sauce for fruit.

Makes 25 servings, ¼ cup each.

Per Serving: 46 Calories

Protein 2 gr.	Carb. 9 gr.
Fat 0 gr.	Cal. from fat 0%
Chol. 0 mg.	Sodium 28 mg.

Strawberry Sauce

1 cup fresh strawberries
¼ cup all-fruit strawberry spread

Purée strawberries in blender until smooth. Add fruit spread and mix well.

A delicious dessert sauce or topping for fresh fruit, pancakes or French toast.

Makes 4 servings, ¼ cup each.

Per Serving: 35 Calories

Protein 0 gr.	Carb. 8.5 gr.
Fat 0 gr.	Cal. from fat 0%
Chol. 0 mg.	Sodium 17 mg.

Creative Ways With Fruit Sauces

Fruit sauces can be more than sweet toppings; they can become the crowning touch to your presentation. Buy a ketchup-type squirt bottle and spoon the sauce into it (you may need to thin the sauce with unsweetened white grape juice). Then you can "paint" it on dishes with a plan or with a random, creative squeeze.

You can make a beautiful heart design by squeezing droplets of sauce on the plate, then quickly pulling a toothpick through the sauce. You can also blend sauces together, using the whiter yogurt sauce as the base, and adding drops of fruit sauce on top.

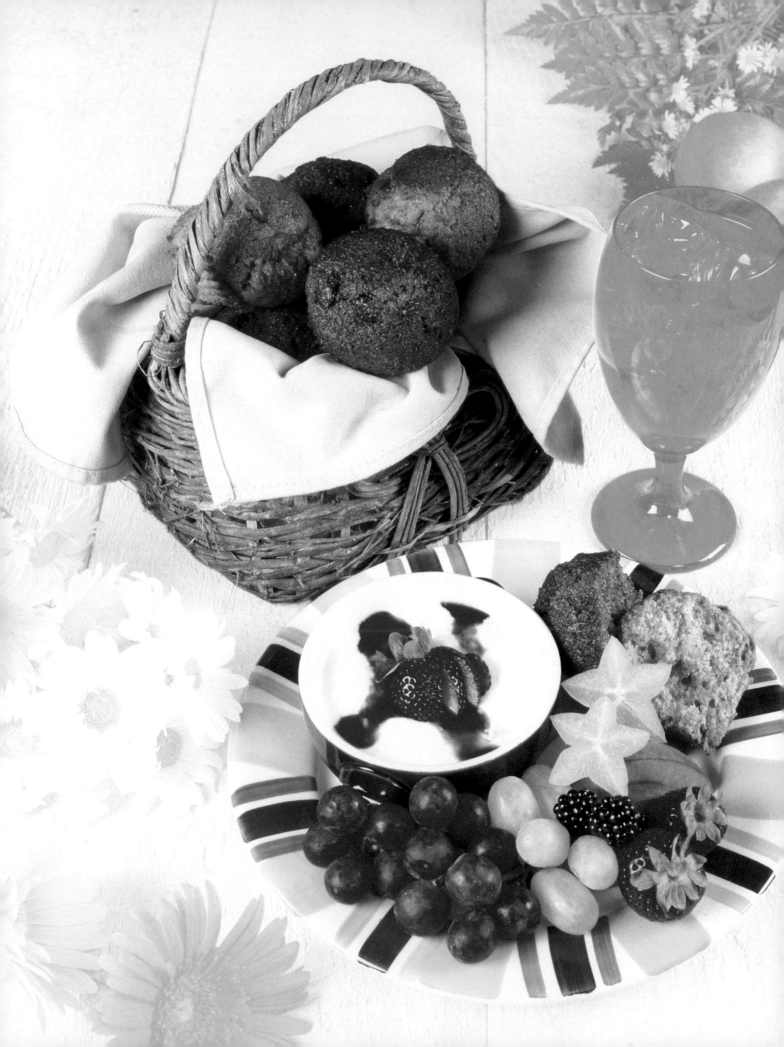

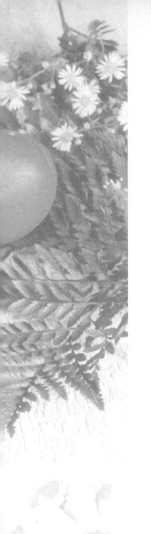

breakfasts
TWENTY-TWO MEALS

Don't let busy mornings keep you from getting the fuel your body needs! Just as Mom always said—breakfast really is vital for peak performance that lasts all day long. It's the perfect start to a day filled with boundless energy and well-being! Breakfast stokes the fire of your metabolism and gets it burning bright and strong. Eating breakfast sets the stage for optimal moods and performance—even clearer thinking and memory!

The key for breakfast is to have it, to have it soon (within half an hour of arising) and to have it balanced. A balanced breakfast supplies adequate carbohydrates and protein.

Don't resort to the food industry's versions of "instant" breakfasts, like toaster fruit pies, granola bars (just candy with oats) and artificially flavored and colored powdered drink mixes. Instead of going for breakfast in the fast lane— and getting much more fat, calories and sodium than you've bargained for—grab and go with your own quick and easy breakfast. Your body will be grateful and will gladly return the favor by working for you rather than working against you.

When you grab coffee and toast, you're depriving your body of the simple carbohydrates and protein it needs to get started. American breakfast favorites focus on the complex carbohydrates (bagels, English muffins, pancakes, muffins and toast) but ignore the rest.

A power breakfast includes some breakfast add-ons. For simple carbohydrate add-ons, choose seasonal fresh fruit in the portion sizes shown on pages 38 and 39. In addition to eggs,

Pictured: Bran and Apple Raisin Muffins (pg. 66–67)

Canadian bacon and low-fat cheese, there are extra-quick proteins you can choose such as skim milk, nonfat yogurt and nonfat cream cheese. Their nutritional analyses are as follows.

SKIM MILK: 80 calories per 1 cup serving, 8 gr. protein, 12 gr. carbohydrates, 0 gr. fat, 0% calories from fat, 4 mg. cholesterol, 125 mg. sodium.

NONFAT YOGURT: 120 calories per 1 cup serving, 13 gr. protein, 17 gr. carbohydrates, 0 gr. fat, 0% calories from fat, 4 mg. cholesterol, 174 mg. sodium.

NONFAT CREAM CHEESE: 20 calories per 2 Tbsp. serving, 3 gr. protein, 2 gr. carbohydrate, 0 gr. fat, 0% calories from fat, 15 mg. cholesterol, 150 mg. sodium.

The recipes on the following pages are just a few of the many ways you can get your morning—and your metabolism—off to a terrific start. I take many of our traditional favorites and reduce the fat while powering up the flavor. I also introduce you to some treats you may not have tried before, including grits and a very special yogurt parfait.

Muffins

Bran Muffins

skim milk or yogurt (protein)
muffin (complex carb.)
raisins (simple carb.)

¼ cup unprocessed wheat bran
¼ cup unprocessed oat bran
⅓ cup boiling water
½ cup milk
3 Tbsp. packed brown sugar
3 Tbsp. canola oil
3 Tbsp. honey
4 egg whites (or ½ cup egg substitute)
1 ⅓ cups whole-wheat pastry flour
2 tsp. baking powder
1 tsp. cinnamon
¼ tsp. salt
½ cup raisins

───────────

● Serve with 8 oz. yogurt or skim milk per serving.

Preheat oven to 400 degrees.

Spray the bottoms in a 12-well muffin tin with cooking spray or line with paper baking cups.

Mix brans and boiling water; set aside. In medium bowl, beat milk, brown sugar, oil, honey and egg whites. Add bran mixture, flour, baking powder, cinnamon and salt; stir until moistened (batter will be lumpy). Fold in raisins.

Divide batter evenly among muffin cups. Cups will be about two-thirds full. Bake 20 to 25 minutes or until golden brown. Immediately remove from pan.

Makes 12 muffins, 1 per serving.

Per Serving: 138 Calories

Protein 4 gr.	Carb. 24 gr.
Fat 3 gr.	Cal. from fat 23%
Chol. 0 mg.	Sodium 71 mg.

Pumpkin-Spice Muffins

cheese spread (protein)
muffin (complex carb.)
pumpkin, apricots (simple carb.)

2 cups whole-wheat pastry flour
3 Tbsp. packed brown sugar
1 tsp. cinnamon
1 tsp. pumpkin pie spice
¼ tsp. salt
½ tsp. baking soda
2 tsp. baking powder
⅔ cup canned pumpkin
1 cup evaporated skim milk
3 Tbsp. canola oil
2 Tbsp. honey
2 egg whites (or ¼ cup egg substitute)

───────────

● Serve with 2 Tbsp. Apricot Cheese Spread (pg. 67) per serving.

Preheat oven to 400 degrees.

Spray the bottoms in a 12-well muffin tin with cooking spray or line with paper baking cups.

Mix flour, sugar, spices, salt, baking soda and baking powder in a bowl. In another bowl whisk together pumpkin, evaporated milk, oil, honey and egg whites. Add pumpkin mixture to dry ingredients and stir until just moistened (batter will be lumpy).

Divide batter evenly among muffin cups. Cups will be about two-thirds full. Bake 20 to 25 minutes or until golden brown. Immediately remove from pan and place on wire rack to cool.

Makes 12 muffins, 1 per serving.

Per Serving: 146 Calories

Protein 5 gr.	Carb. 24 gr.
Fat 3 gr.	Cal. from fat 23%
Chol. 0 mg.	Sodium 80 mg.

Taking the Fat Out of Muffins

Removing fat from muffins, quick breads and other baked goods often leaves them with a rubbery texture. Fortunately, you can overcome this by replacing the fat with fruit or puréed vegetables like pumpkin. The fruit's pectin prevents moisture loss during baking.

Lower-fat muffins will also retain their moisture better when baked in large 3-inch muffin cups.

You can bake enough of these high-fiber low-fat muffins for 2 weeks. Store in sealable plastic freezer bags and heat in microwave or toaster oven as needed.

Muffins (continued)

Apple-Raisin Muffins

cheese spread, skim milk or yogurt (protein)
muffin (complex carb.)
raisins, apples (simple carb.)

2 large egg whites
1/3 cup maple syrup
3 Tbsp. unsweetened white grape juice
1 cup skim milk
1 Tbsp. vanilla extract
1 tsp. cinnamon
1 tsp. allspice
1/2 tsp. ground cloves
1/4 tsp. salt
1 1/2 cups rolled oats
1 cup whole-wheat pastry flour
1 tsp. baking powder
1/4 cup pecans, chopped
1 cup peeled and chopped apples
1/4 cup golden raisins

- Serve with your choice of Date Cheese Spread, Apricot Cheese Spread or 8 oz. yogurt or skim milk per serving.

Preheat oven to 350 degrees.

Spray the bottoms in a 12-well muffin tin with cooking spray or line with paper baking cups.

Put the egg whites in a large mixing bowl and whisk until frothy. Whisk in the syrup, juice and milk. Add the vanilla, spices and salt. Stir in the oats, flour and baking powder. Fold in the pecans, apples and raisins.

Divide batter evenly among muffin cups. Cups will be about two-thirds full. Bake for about 20 minutes or until the muffins are firm in the center.

Makes 12 muffins, 1 per serving.

Per Serving: 128 Calories

Protein 4.5 gr.	Carb. 23 gr.
Fat 2.4 gr.	Cal. from fat 16%
Chol. 0 mg.	Sodium 94 mg.

Date Cheese Spread

2 pkgs. (8 oz. each) fat-free or light cream cheese
8 oz. unsweetened pitted dates, chopped
2 Tbsp. skim milk
1/2 cup walnuts, chopped

Process all ingredients in a food processor or blender until mixed evenly. Transfer to airtight container and store in refrigerator for up to 2 weeks.

Serving size: 3 Tbsp.

Per Serving: 64 Calories

Protein 4 gr.	Carb. 12 gr.
Fat 1 gr.	Cal. from fat 14%
Chol. 15 mg.	Sodium 151 mg.

Apricot Cheese Spread

1 pkg. (8 oz.) fat-free cream cheese, softened
1/4 cup apricot all-fruit spread

In a bowl, blend cream cheese and all-fruit spread. Store in refrigerator for up to 4 weeks.

Makes about 1 1/4 cups, 2 Tbsp. per serving.

Per Serving: 40 Calories

Protein 3 gr.	Carb. 7 gr.
Fat 0 gr.	Cal. from fat 0%
Chol. 15 mg.	Sodium 150 mg.

Tips for Lighter Muffins

- *Substituting buttermilk or yogurt for milk in muffin batter will yield light, tender muffins; just add 1/2 tsp. baking soda for each cup of buttermilk or yogurt used.*

- *If a muffin recipe calls for whole eggs, separating them will make the muffin lighter. Mix the yolks with the other moist ingredients; beat the whites until stiff and fold them in after the rest of ingredients are combined.*

- *Stirring muffin batter too vigorously creates tough muffins. Stir the batter only until all the dry ingredients are moistened, leaving it lumpy.*

Great Granola and Cereal

Healthy Living Granola

⅓ cup dried apricots
⅔ cup dried pears, peaches or apples
⅓ cup golden raisins
3 cups old-fashioned oats
⅓ cup pumpkin seeds, shelled
⅓ cup sunflower seed kernels
1 cup unsweetened coconut milk
1 cup unsweetened prune juice

Preheat oven to 350 degrees.

Dice fruits into ¼-inch bits. Toss with oats and seeds. Set aside.

In a saucepan, combine the coconut milk and prune juice. Over low heat, reduce juices to 1 cup (½ their original volume). This should take about 20 to 25 minutes. Mix juices with oat mixture. Spread into a shallow pan. Bake for 15 to 20 minutes, stirring every 5 minutes, until golden brown. Break into pieces and cool uncovered. Store in an airtight container.

This granola may be used in many of my breakfast meals, or may be sprinkled over fruit or yogurt as a crunchy dessert.

Makes 8 cups, ½ cup per serving.

Per Serving: 145 Calories

Protein 4.4 gr.	Carb. 30 gr.
Fat 4 gr.	Cal. from fat 23%
Chol. 0 mg.	Sodium 3 mg.

Granola Breakfast

milk, seeds (protein)
oats (complex carb.)
fruits, juices (simple carb.)

½ cup Healthy Living Granola
2 sliced strawberries
¼ banana, sliced
2 Tbsp. blueberries
¾ cup skim milk or nonfat yogurt

Combine all in a bowl and enjoy.
Serves 1.

Per Serving: 247 Calories

Protein 11 gr.	Carb. 43 gr.
Fat 4 gr.	Cal. from fat 14%
Chol. 3 mg.	Sodium 98 mg.

Whole-Grain Cereal With Berries

skim milk (protein)
cereal (complex carb.)
strawberries (simple carb.)

1 oz. (about ¾ cup) any whole-grain cereal (list of cereals on pg. 36)
½ cup sliced strawberries
1 cup skim milk

Pour cereal into bowl. Top with sliced strawberries and skim milk.
Serves 1.

Per Serving: 227 Calories

Protein 11 gr.	Carb. 45 gr.
Fat 1 gr.	Cal. from fat 4%
Chol. 4 mg.	Sodium 351 mg.

Granola Alternatives?

Granola typically contains lots of fat from the oil, nuts and seeds, and is often loaded with sweeteners and honey. Why not try a great-tasting, great-for-you alternative?

Say Yes to Yogurt

The health benefits of yogurt have long been touted. It's a good source of B vitamins, protein and calcium, and is much more digestible than fresh milk. It keeps the intestinal system populated with good bacteria (acidophilus and lactobacillus) and therefore healthy. Unfortunately, frozen yogurt doesn't have the same promise! Buy nonfat plain yogurt or fruit-flavored yogurt (sweetened with juice, preferably with no sugar added).

You may store yogurt in the refrigerator for up to 10 days after the carton date.

Cool Starts

Freshly Fruited Yogurt Parfait

yogurt (protein)
granola (complex carb.)
fruit (simple carb.)

1/4 cup low-fat granola (purchased or
   Healthy Living Granola, pg. 68)
2 Tbsp. blueberries
4 strawberries, sliced
1/2 banana, sliced
1 cup nonfat plain yogurt
1 Tbsp. all-fruit spread

Crunch 1 Tbsp. of granola into the bottom of a parfait glass. Top with 2 sliced strawberries, 1 Tbsp. blueberries and half of the banana slices.

Mix the yogurt with the all-fruit spread; spoon half of yogurt mixture atop the fruit, then sprinkle with 2 Tbsp. granola. Top with the remaining strawberries, blueberries and bananas, and the rest of the yogurt mixture. Sprinkle with final 1 Tbsp. granola.

Other fresh seasonal berries may be used in place of strawberries and blueberries. Good choices are raspberries and blackberries.

Serves 1.

Per Serving: 246 Calories

Protein 15 gr.	Carb. 41 gr.
Fat 2 gr.	Cal. from fat 7%
Chol. 4 mg.	Sodium 195 mg.

Fresh Fruit Shake

yogurt (protein)
bread (complex carb.)
fruit (simple carb.)

1/2 cup ice cubes
1/2 cup fresh berries
1/2 banana
1/2 cup orange juice
1 cup nonfat plain yogurt
2 tsp. honey
1 tsp. vanilla

_____

• Serve with 1 slice of toast or 1/2 English muffin.

Place ice into a blender, cover and crush. Add fruit and blend until smooth. Add remaining ingredients and blend until mixed well.
   Serves 2.

Per Serving: 150 Calories

Protein 7.5 gr.	Carb. 30 gr.
Fat less than 1 gr.	Cal. from fat 3%
Chol. 2 mg.	Sodium 88 mg.

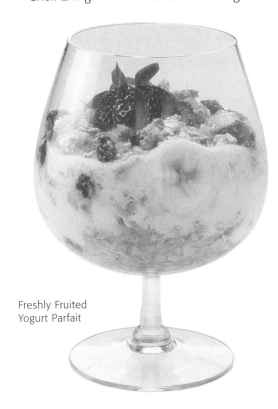

Freshly Fruited
Yogurt Parfait

Fruit Shake Breakfasts— in an Instant

• *Make your own "instant breakfast" by assembling fruit shake ingredients (except the ice cubes) in a blender before bed; cover and refrigerate. All you have to do the next morning is add crushed ice and push the blender button to create this delicious jump-start to your day!*

• *Do your bananas ripen quicker than you can eat them? Freeze them whole and in their skin. (They'll turn black as molasses, but they'll be fine.) You can also freeze in-season ripe peaches or berries in zip-top freezer bags. These will make your fruit shake quick, easy and great!*

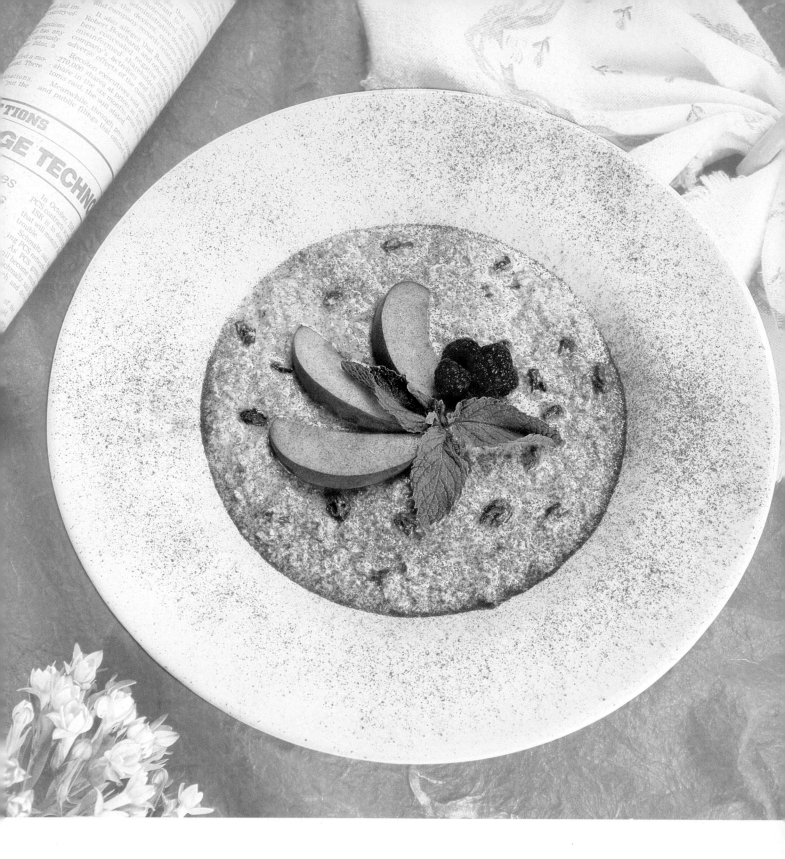

A steaming bowl of apple-scented oatmeal perfectly spiced with cinnamon and raisins can warm you down to your toes—and supply you with wholesome fiber, essential nutrients and stick-to-the-ribs satisfaction. Oatmeal can be cooked quickly in the microwave or gently on the stove. Either will get your day started in a smart way!

Morning Warm-Ups

Cinnamon Raisin Oatmeal

skim milk (protein)
oats (complex carb.)
juice, raisins (simple carb.)

²⁄₃ cup quick oatmeal
1 cup skim milk
½ cup unsweetened white grape juice
    or apple juice
2 Tbsp. raisins, dark or golden
½ tsp. cinnamon
1 tsp. vanilla extract

In a microwave-safe bowl, stir together oatmeal, skim milk and juice. Microwave on high, covered with plastic wrap and vented, for 4 minutes or until it reaches desired thickness. Stir in raisins, cinnamon and vanilla, and serve.
  Serves 2.

Per Serving: 206 Calories

Protein 9 gr.	Carb. 39 gr.
Fat 2 gr.	Cal. from fat 9%
Chol. 2 mg.	Sodium 65 mg.

Nicole's Cheesy Hash Browns

cheese (protein)
potatoes (complex carb.)
melon (simple carb.)

1 bag Simply Potatoes shredded hash
  browns
1 tsp. Mrs. Dash seasoning
½ tsp. creole seasoning
1 cup grated part-skim cheddar cheese
1 Tbsp. chopped fresh herbs (cilantro,
  basil, rosemary, thyme)

- Serve with ¼ melon, sliced.

Spray nonstick skillet with cooking spray; heat. Empty hash browns into pan and add seasonings. Allow bottom of potatoes to brown lightly, then flip over in sections until all are browned and crisp. Sprinkle with chopped herbs. Top with grated cheese and let melt.
  Serves 4.

Per Serving: 298 Calories

Protein 10 gr.	Carb. 39 mg.
Fat 4.5 gr.	Cal. from fat 18%
Chol. 18 mg.	Sodium 282 mg.

Fiber Facts

There are two types of fibers: soluble and nonsoluble. Soluble fibers are found in apples, dried beans, peanuts, barley and oat bran.

These fibers have been found to lower both triglycerides and cholesterol, and they help control blood sugars.

The nonsoluble fibers are found in wheat bran, whole-grain breads, cereals, fruits and vegetables. They are an excellent means of controlling digestive challenges.

You need both soluble and nonsoluble fiber and lots of wonderful water to keep your body working at its best!

Skillet Breakfasts

Sweet Pepper Frittata

egg substitute, egg whites (protein)
potatoes (complex carb.)
oranges, vegetables (simple carb.)

4 small red-skinned potatoes, cut into
   quarters
1 tsp. olive oil
½ each red and yellow bell peppers,
   sliced thin lengthwise
1 small onion, diced
1 clove garlic, minced
1 tsp. Mrs. Dash seasoning
½ tsp. creole seasoning
1 tomato, seeded and chopped
1 cup egg substitute (or 4 large eggs)
4 large egg whites
¼ cup grated Parmesan cheese

———————

● Serve with 3 oranges, cut into quarters.

Place potatoes in a microwaveable bowl with ¼ cup water; cover with plastic wrap and vent. Microwave on high for 5 to 6 minutes or until potatoes begin to get tender. Drain.

Preheat oven broiler. Spray a large, ovenproof nonstick skillet with cooking spray. Add olive oil and heat on the stove to medium-high heat. Add peppers, onion, garlic, seasonings and half of the tomato. Cook, stirring, until the onions are limp, about 4 minutes. Add the microwaved potatoes.

In a bowl whisk together the egg substitute, egg whites and Parmesan cheese, and pour into the skillet, gently stirring to distribute the vegetables. Cook over low heat until the underside is light golden, about 5 minutes.

Place the skillet under the broiler and broil until the top of the frittata is puffed and golden brown, 1 to 2 minutes. Loosen the frittata and slide onto a platter. Cut into 4 wedges and sprinkle with remaining tomatoes. Add 3 wedges of orange to each serving.

Serves 4.

Per Serving: 167 Calories

Protein 11 gr.	Carb. 25 gr.
Fat 2.5 gr.	Cal. from fat 14%
Chol. 4 mg.	Sodium 282 mg.

Huevos Rancheros

egg substitute, beans (protein)
tortilla, beans (complex carb.)
salsa, melon (simple carb.)

1 burrito-sized, fat-free flour tortilla
¼ cup black beans, cooked and
   drained
¼ cup chicken stock (fat-free/low salt)
¼ tsp. creole seasoning, divided
1 tsp. Mrs. Dash seasoning, divided
½ cup egg substitute (or 2 large eggs)
¼ cup tomato salsa (purchased)

———————

● Serve with ¼ cantaloupe, sliced.

Spray tortilla with nonstick cooking spray. Place into heated nonstick skillet and grill until crisp. Set aside.

Spray skillet with cooking spray. Add black beans, chicken stock, ⅛ tsp. creole seasoning and ½ tsp. of Mrs. Dash; sauté until beans are easily mashed. Spread black bean mixture on tortilla.

Spray skillet with cooking spray again; add egg substitute and remaining seasonings. Scramble. Spoon on top of beans and top with salsa.

Serves 1.

Per Serving: 200 Calories

Protein 14 gr.	Carb. 38 gr.
Fat 1 gr.	Cal. from fat 5%
Chol. 0 mg.	Sodium 599 mg.

**Are Eggs Good
for You?**

Eggs have been given a bad rap and for somewhat of a good reason. It's true that one egg gives 71 percent of all the cholesterol the average person needs in one day. Yet up-to-date studies have shown that eggs are not the culprit. The highly saturated fat in other breakfast foods such as bacon, sausage and butter is the real enemy. It converts to the bad form of cholesterol in the body. Next time, hold the bacon!

Grits: A Southern Specialty

Cheese Grits Pie

cheese, turkey bacon (protein)
grits (complex carb.)
strawberries (simple carb.)

3/4 cup grated Jarlsberg Lite cheese
4 cups cooked grits
2 Tbsp. chopped fresh parsley
1 tsp. Mrs. Dash seasoning
1 tsp. creole seasoning

___

- Serve with 1 pt. strawberries, washed and hulled, and 8 slices turkey bacon, microwaved.

Mix cheese, grits, parsley and seasonings, and pour into a sheet pan sprayed with cooking spray. Refrigerate until firm; cut into 8 squares. In nonstick skillet sprayed with cooking spray, brown the squares over medium to medium-high heat until lightly browned and crisp. Place 2 squares on plate with 5 sliced strawberries and 2 slices turkey bacon.
Serves 4.

Per Serving: 286 Calories

Protein 13.5 gr.	Carb. 40 gr.
Fat 8 gr.	Cal. from fat 25%
Chol. 32 mg.	Sodium 747 mg.

Get-Going Grits

cheese (protein)
grits (complex carb.)
apple (simple carb.)

1 tsp. canola oil
2 Tbsp. minced onions
1 small green bell pepper, seeded and finely chopped
2 medium tomatoes, peeled and coarsely chopped
3 drops hot pepper sauce
3 cups water
1/2 tsp. creole seasoning
3/4 cup quick-cooking grits
1 1/2 cups grated part-skim sharp cheddar cheese

___

- Serve with 1 apple per serving, cut into wedges.

Spray a medium-sized nonstick skillet with cooking spray. Add canola oil and heat over medium-high heat. Add onion and green pepper and sauté until tender. Stir in tomatoes and hot pepper sauce. Reduce heat and simmer uncovered 20 minutes or until thickened. Set aside.
Combine water and seasoning in medium saucepan; bring to a boil. Stir in grits. Cover, reduce heat and simmer 5 minutes or until thickened, stirring occasionally. Stir in grated cheese and remove from heat; stir in tomato mixture. Serve immediately with apple wedges.
Serves 6.

Per Serving: 232 Calories

Protein 8 gr.	Carb. 40 gr.
Fat 5 gr.	Cal. from fat 20%
Chol. 13 mg.	Sodium 203 mg.

Grits Are Great

If you've never tried grits before, you're in for a treat. This Southern favorite will add a dash of variety to your breakfast menus.

You can prepare grits simply, according to the package directions, as a delicious side dish for eggs or lean meats. Or, try these cheese grits recipes and see why grits are called "Georgia ice cream"!

Omelettes

Egg White Omelette

egg whites (protein)
bran muffin (complex carb.)
berries, sauce (simple carb.)

3 egg whites
1 Tbsp. white wine*
2 tsp. chopped chives
½ tsp. Mrs. Dash seasoning
¼ tsp. creole seasoning
2 strawberries, quartered
2 Tbsp. blueberries
2 Tbsp. Strawberry Sauce (pg. 63)

* or substitute dealcoholized wine or
chicken stock (fat-free/low salt)

———————————

- Serve with 1 warmed Bran Muffin
  (pg. 66).

Whip egg whites halfway stiff. Stir in wine,
chives and seasonings. Spray a 12-inch nonstick
skillet with cooking spray. Heat skillet on very
low heat; add egg white mixture. Cook on very
low heat until mixture stiffens on bottom. With
spatula, carefully turn over like a pancake. Finish
cooking, and fold to make an omelette.

Drizzle with strawberry sauce and fresh
berries.

Serves 1.

Per Serving: 116 Calories

Protein 11 gr.	Carb. 17 gr.
Fat less than 1 gr.	Cal. from fat 0%
Chol. 0 mg.	Sodium 467 mg.

Garden Omelette

egg substitute (protein)
English muffin (complex carb.)
strawberries, vegetables (simple carb.)

½ tomato, seeded and diced
2 medium mushrooms, diced
½ green onion, sliced
½ cup egg substitute (or 2 large eggs)
1 tsp. Mrs. Dash seasoning
¼ tsp. creole seasoning

———————————

- Serve with ½ English muffin,
  toasted, and 5 strawberries.

Spray a nonstick skillet with cooking spray.
Heat on medium heat. Add tomato, mushroom
and onion; quickly sauté until tender.

Whip egg substitute with seasonings, and
pour into pan with vegetables. Cook both sides,
folding to make an omelette.

Serves 1.

Per Serving: 188 Calories

Protein 18 gr.	Carb. 26 gr.
Fat 1 gr.	Cal. from fat 5%
Chol. 0 mg.	Sodium 705 mg.

Egg Substitutions

*Cholesterol-free egg
substitutes can be used
in cooking and baking
in many (though
not all) of the same
ways as regular eggs.
Egg substitutes are egg
whites mixed with beta
carotene for color. They
also contain a touch of
natural coagulant
derived from seaweed.
Vitamins and minerals
are added to boost
nutrition.*

*You can also replace
whole eggs (although
loaded with nutrients,
they are also loaded
with fat) with no-fat,
no-cholesterol, pure
protein egg whites. Just
use 2 egg whites (¼
cup) for one whole egg
in cooking.*

*You can easily separate
cold eggs by cracking
them into a wire mesh
strainer over a mixing
bowl. The white will drip
through the strainer's
holes into the bowl, and
the yolk will remain in
the strainer.*

Cheese Delights

Fiesta Cheese Cloud

cheese, eggs, milk, bacon (protein)
bread (complex carb.)
strawberries (simple carb.)

12 slices whole-wheat bread
½ lb. turkey bacon, chopped
2 Tbsp. grated red onion
2 cloves garlic, minced
8 oz. grated part-skim mozzarella/
   part-skim cheddar cheese blend
1 cup egg substitute (or 4 eggs)
2½ cups skim milk
1 Tbsp. Dijon mustard
½ tsp. creole seasoning
1 tsp. Mrs. Dash seasoning
1 small can of green chilies, chopped

- Serve with ½ cup sliced strawberries per serving.

Preheat oven to 325 degrees.

Trim crusts from bread cut in half into triangular shapes. Arrange 12 of the triangles in bottom of a 12- x 8-inch greased baking dish.

In a nonstick skillet, sauté bacon until crisp. Remove from pan and drain on paper towel. Add onion and garlic to pan, and sauté until transparent.

Sprinkle turkey bacon and half of grated cheese onto bread slices in pan, then top with sautéed onion and garlic. Add remaining bread slices.

Beat eggs; add milk, mustard and seasonings; add chilies (with liquid). Pour liquid over casserole and let stand at room temperature for 1 hour (or even refrigerate overnight if more convenient). Bake 1 hour; serve immediately.

Serves 8.

Per Serving: 249 Calories

Protein 22 gr.	Carb. 23 gr.
Fat 7 gr.	Cal. from fat 17%
Chol. 39 mg.	Sodium 545 mg.

Turkey Bacon and Cheese Biscuits

turkey bacon, cheese (protein)
biscuit (complex carb.)
cantaloupe (simple carb.)

1 can purchased low-fat biscuits
3 slices turkey bacon, halved
¾ cup grated part-skim cheddar/
   fat-free mozzarella cheese blend

- Serve with ¼ cantaloupe, sliced, per serving.

Bake biscuits according to package directions. While biscuits are baking, place turkey bacon slices on a plate lined with paper towels, and microwave for 3 minutes or until crisp. Or, brown and crisp bacon in a nonstick skillet.

When biscuits are done, slice each open partway, add ½ slice of bacon and sprinkle with 1 Tbsp. grated cheese. Put back into hot oven for 1 to 2 minutes or until cheese melts.

Makes 3 servings, 2 biscuits each.

Per Serving: 206 Calories

Protein 11 gr.	Carb. 27 gr.
Fat 6 gr.	Cal. from fat 26%
Chol. 18 mg.	Sodium 415 mg.

Treat Yourself to Turkey Bacon

Turkey bacon is a new product that serves well the occasional desire for this popular breakfast meat. It has less than half the fat of traditional bacon, yet contains more protein.

To microwave bacon, line a microwaveable rack or paper plate with a double layer of microwaveable paper towels. Place strips side by side and cover with another paper towel. Six slices cooked on high will take about 3 to 4 minutes.

The sodium and nitrate content is still present in turkey bacon, so don't make this a daily treat!

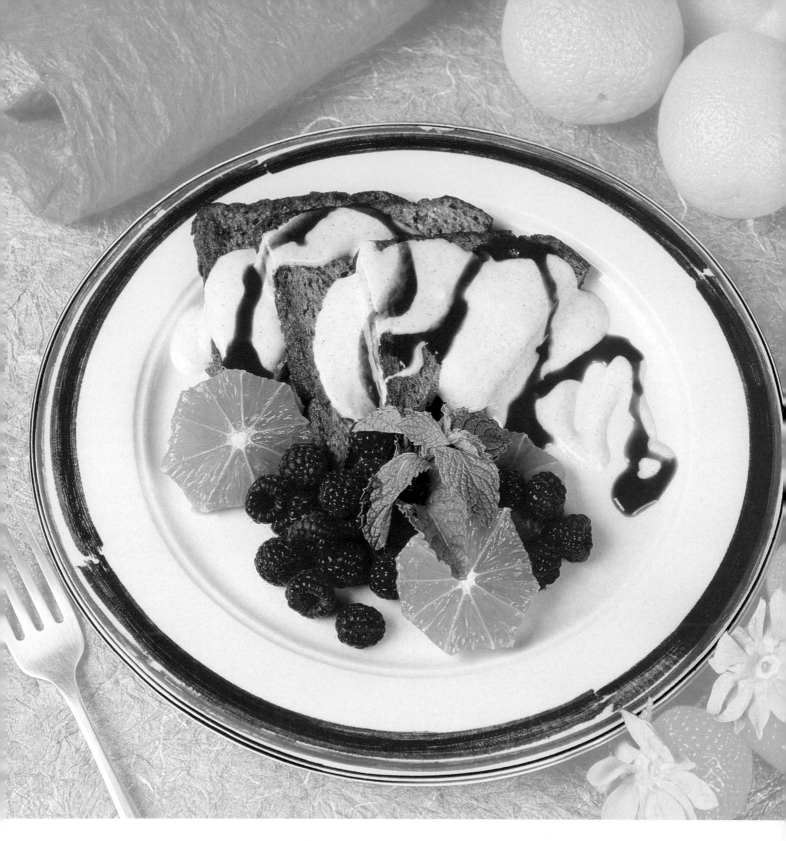

This breakfast can be a sunshiny start to your day—simple and quick to make, yet deliciously satisfying. The orange and vanilla flavorings are a perfect complement to yogurt sauce and berry topping—and any in-season fruit makes for a perfect garnish. Try tripling this recipe for future breakfasts—freeze individual slices in zip-top bags for a toast-'n-go breakfast.

Favorites Without the Fat

Country French Toast

eggs, milk (protein)
bread (complex carb.)
fruit, fruit sauce (simple carb.)

¼ cup orange juice
½ cup skim milk
4 egg whites, lightly beaten
2 tsp. vanilla
1 tsp. cinnamon
6 slices whole-wheat bread
1 cup Yogurt Fruit Sauce (pg. 63)

⎯⎯⎯⎯⎯⎯

• Serve with ¼ cup Strawberry Sauce (pg. 63) and ¼ cup fresh berries per serving.

In a medium-sized dish, whisk together juice, milk, egg whites, vanilla and cinnamon. Add bread slices, one at a time, allowing to soak in egg mixture. Let sit for 4 to 5 minutes.

Spray a nonstick skillet or griddle with cooking spray. Heat. With spatula, gently lift bread slices onto heated surface and brown on both sides. When done, cut toast into triangles and place 3 triangles on each plate; top with ¼ cup Yogurt Fruit Sauce, then drizzle plate with 2 Tbsp. Strawberry Sauce and garnish with berries.

Makes 4 servings, 1½ slices of bread each.

Per Serving: 286 Calories

Protein 13 gr.	Carb. 56 gr.
Fat 2 gr.	Cal. from fat 7%
Chol. 1.5 mg.	Sodium 416 mg.

Cinnamon Apple Puff Pancakes

eggs (protein)
pancakes (complex carb.)
apples (simple carb.)

1 cup whole-wheat pastry flour
1 tsp. baking powder
½ tsp. salt
1½ cups egg substitute (or 5 eggs)
1 cup skim milk
2 tsp. canola oil
3 cups fresh apples, sliced
1 Tbsp. honey
juice of ½ lemon
1 tsp. ground cinnamon

Preheat oven to 425 degrees.

In a medium bowl, mix together flour, baking powder and salt. In another bowl, beat eggs with wire whisk; whisk in milk. Pour into dry ingredients and blend until moistened.

Coat a 12-inch ovenproof skillet with cooking spray. Spread oil over bottom of skillet and heat over medium heat until water droplets "dance" over bottom. Pour all batter into skillet and cook for 1 minute. Transfer skillet to oven and bake uncovered for 20 minutes until pancake is golden and puffy.

While pancake is baking, spray a nonstick skillet with cooking spray; heat. Add apples and quickly sauté with honey, lemon juice and cinnamon until tender and syrupy.

When pancake is done, remove from oven and spread with apples. Slice into 4 wedges to serve.

Makes 4 servings.

Per Serving: 231 Calories

Protein 11 gr.	Carb. 42 gr.
Fat 3 gr.	Cal. from fat 10%
Chol. 1 mg.	Sodium 476 mg.

Choose Whole-Wheat Flour

Whole-wheat flour is a light brown flour that has the nutty taste of the grain. It has a higher fiber and nutritional content than all-purpose or bread flour because it's milled from the whole kernel and contains the germ.

Whole-wheat pastry flour is the best choice for muffins, pancakes or waffles because it is more finely milled from a soft wheat. If not available, use a blend of unbleached white and regular whole wheat.

Pancakes

Pancake Lover Tips

To make fluffy pancakes, only mix the ingredients together until moistened, yet still lumpy. Beating till smooth will make rubber tires!

Most pancake batters can be covered and refrigerated overnight to save precious morning time. If the batter thickens too much, add 1 to 2 Tbsp. skim milk. If it's more than a day old, add 1/4 tsp. more baking powder along with the cold milk.

Use 1/4-cup measure of batter to make a 5-inch pancake. Make sure your skillet is very hot before pouring in the batter.

Quick-Mix Pancakes

milk or yogurt (protein)
pancake (complex carb.)
fruit topping (simple carb.)

1 3/4 cups Homemade Pancake Mix
1 cup water (or club soda to make pancakes even lighter)
2 egg whites (or 1/4 cup egg substitute), beaten
1 Tbsp. honey

_____

- Serve with 1 cup skim milk or yogurt and 1/4 cup Pourable Fruit (pg. 79) per serving.

Combine pancake mix, water, egg whites and honey; stir gently until completely moistened. Drop by quarter-cupfuls onto a hot nonstick skillet sprayed with cooking spray. Cook until bottoms are lightly browned. Flip and cook until bottoms are set.

Freeze any leftovers in individual freezer bags. When ready to use, toast to thaw and heat.

Makes 6 servings, 2 pancakes per serving.

Per Serving: 284 Calories

Protein 11.5 gr.	Carb. 49 gr.
Fat 7 gr.	Cal. from fat 22%
Chol. 15 mg.	Sodium 586 mg.

Homemade Pancake Mix

4 cups whole-wheat pastry flour
1 tsp. salt
1 cup nonfat dry milk powder
2 1/2 Tbsp. baking powder
1/4 cup canola oil

Mix flour, salt, dry milk and baking powder. Slowly pour in oil, mixing until completely moistened. May be stored in the refrigerator for up to 6 weeks. Use to make Quick Mix Pancakes.

Whole-Wheat Waffles

egg white, buttermilk (protein)
flour (complex carb.)
fruit topping (simple carb.)

2 cups whole-wheat pastry flour
1 tsp. baking powder
1/2 tsp. baking soda
1/4 tsp. ground cinnamon
2 1/2 cups low-fat buttermilk
1 tsp. honey
1 tsp. vanilla
3 egg whites

_____

- Serve with 1/4 cup Strawberry Sauce (pg. 63) or Pourable Fruit (pg. 79) per serving.

Combine first four ingredients in a bowl; stir well. Mix the buttermilk, honey and vanilla in a separate bowl; add to the dry ingredients, stirring until the dry ingredients are moistened.

Beat egg whites with mixer at high speed until soft peaks form. Gently fold them into mixture.

Coat a waffle iron with cooking spray; heat. Spoon 1/3 cup of batter per waffle onto hot waffle iron, spreading batter to edges. Cook 5 minutes or until the steaming stops. Repeat with remaining batter. Place finished waffles on a large baking sheet (lined with a dish towel) in a single layer and hold in 200-degree oven until ready to serve.

Makes 6 servings, 2 waffles each.

Per Serving: 138 Calories

Protein 8 gr.	Carb. 26 gr.
Fat less than 1 gr.	Cal. from fat 0%
Chol. 1 mg.	Sodium 155 mg.

Pancakes (continued)

Canadian bacon (protein)
pancakes (complex carb.)
fruit topping (simple carb.)

Danny's Perfect Pancakes

2 cups whole-wheat pastry flour
2 tsp. baking soda
1/2 tsp. salt
3/4 cup orange juice
3/4 cup buttermilk
2 egg whites, lightly beaten
1 tsp. vanilla

_____

- Serve with 2 Tbsp. Pourable Fruit or Fruited Yogurt Topping (or use purchased all-fruit syrup) and 1 oz. Canadian bacon per serving.

Measure flour, baking soda and salt into medium-sized bowl. Make a well in the center of mixture. Combine juice, buttermilk, egg whites and vanilla; add to well in center of dry ingredients and stir until just moistened.

For each pancake, pour 1/4 cup batter onto hot griddle or nonstick skillet sprayed with cooking spray. Turn pancakes when tops are covered with bubbles and edges look cooked.

While pancakes are cooking, lay Canadian bacon on a plate lined with paper towels and microwave on high for 2 1/4 minutes or until edges curl. Place on plate with 2 pancakes; drizzle pancakes with 2 Tbsp. Pourable Fruit or Fruited Yogurt Topping.

Makes 6 servings, 2 pancakes each.

Per Serving: 262 Calories

Protein 16 gr.	Carb. 46 gr.
Fat 2.5 gr.	Cal. from fat 8%
Chol. 27 mg.	Sodium 55 mg.

Pourable Fruit

4 cups cut-up fresh, ripe fruit (strawberries, bananas, berries, peaches)
1 cup unsweetened apple juice
1/4 cup water
2 Tbsp. cornstarch
1 Tbsp. lemon juice

Blend fresh fruit and apple juice in blender until smooth. Pour into small saucepan and simmer for 5 minutes. Mix cornstarch with water and lemon juice; add to fruit mixture. Simmer until thick. Refrigerate. This fruit will keep in the refrigerator for up to 5 days.

Makes 4 cups, 1/4 cup per serving.

Per Serving: 19 Calories

Protein 0 gr.	Carb. 4.5 gr.
Fat 0 gr.	Cal. from fat 0%
Chol. 0 mg.	Sodium 1 mg.

Fruited Yogurt Topping

1 cup nonfat plain yogurt
1/4 cup fruit (or 2 Tbsp. all-fruit spread)
ground cinnamon to taste

Combine all ingredients, mixing well. Makes 6 servings, 1/4 cup per serving.

Per Serving: 26 Calories

Protein 2 gr.	Carb. 4.5 gr.
Fat less than 1 gr.	Cal. from fat 0%
Chol. 0 mg.	Sodium 29 mg.

Terrific Pancake Toppings

Are there pancake toppings beyond maple syrup? Absolutely! Try these:

- *All-fruit spread (sweetened with fruit juices rather than sugar)*
- *Fresh fruit syrup or Pourable Fruit*
- *Bananas blended with cinnamon and orange juice, then warmed*
- *Light or fat-free cream cheese, thinned with all-fruit spread and vanilla*
- *Light cream cheese and fresh fruit*
- *Nonfat cottage cheese and fresh fruit*
- *All-fruit yogurt*
- *Natural peanut butter, thinned with apple juice and warmed*

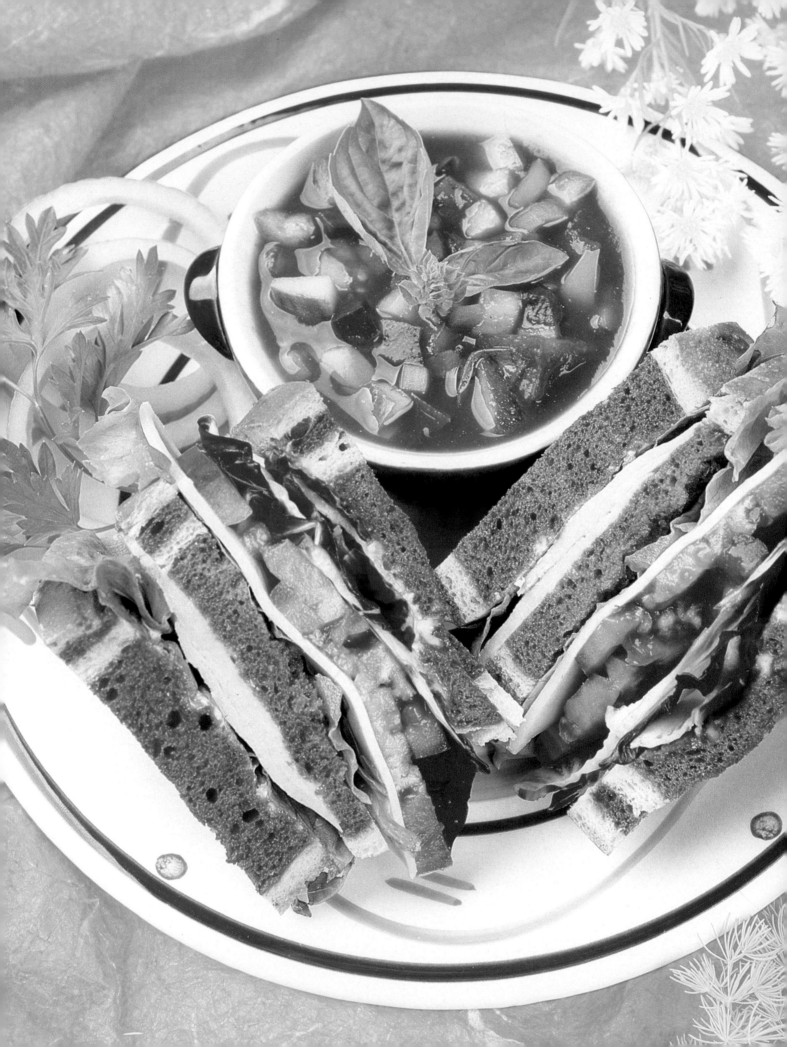

lunches & soups
TWENTY-TWO MEALS

Lunch picks up where breakfast leaves off; it fuels the rest of your day's activities. Like breakfast, lunch should contain a healthy balance of whole grain, complex carbohydrates and low-fat protein to keep your metabolic fires burning brightly and your performance and well-being at their peak. In addition, quick energy-giving, nutrient-filled simple carbohydrates should be part of your lunch in the form of brightly colored fruits and vegetables.

The search for the healthy lunch can be a challenge for many of us because we are at the mercy of the nearest drive-through, cafeteria or restaurant. You don't have much time to grab lunch, let alone think about healthy choices. The temptation is strong to reach for the first appealing thing you see or the "special of the day"—which often turns out not so special at all!

Another option is to pack a lunch. You can do it quickly and be energized with the knowledge that your choice is already made—and it's a smart one.

Be creative with your brown bag lunches. There is life beyond turkey sandwiches—or even peanut butter and jelly!

Pictured: Market Club Sandwich
With Gazpacho (pg. 95)

Breaking the Rut

Whatever you do, try to stay out of the lunchtime rut—it's an easy ditch to fall into—and live in.

We're in a rut when we settle into a limited variety of meals with which we feel safe and don't have to think about much. We don't want to make decisions; it's just easier to have the same things again and again.

The problem with ruts is that we are set up to overindulge as soon as anything more exciting comes along. Once off track, it becomes very difficult to get back on track—since "on track" means returning to the same old, boring rut.

lunches & soups

In addition to the mental reasons ruts are deadly, there are also some nutritional ones. Eating a variety of foods in their whole form provides you with a gamut of vitamins and minerals, including as yet hidden benefits.

Try some of the lunch ideas and recipes that follow to get yourself free from your eating rut and to enjoy a whole new world of food. Think beyond the lunch sandwich altogether—even think beyond bread as the packaging material. Use these guides to help you create your own lunch favorite, possibly in a thermos!

If you make sandwiches in advance, wrap them airtight and refrigerate (they keep for a day that way). You can also freeze meat sandwiches in sandwich bags, then store them in a large freezer-weight bag for up to one month in the freezer. Pull one out of the freezer in the morning, and it will be thawed by lunch. Keep your sandwiches from the soggy blues by packing additions like tomato or pickles in separate plastic bags to tuck in the sandwich just before eating.

Tips for Packing Safety

For safety concerns, how you pack lunch is as important as what you pack. Even the healthiest menu won't prevent the brown-bag bug—food poisoning. Food poisoning symptoms (vomiting, fever, headache, diarrhea and/or stomach cramps) can strike any time from twenty minutes to twenty-four hours after consumption of tainted food.

Lunches carried from home often sit in a desk or locker until noon. That long wait at room temperature makes them a perfect breeding ground for salmonella and other bacteria. The risk of food poisoning soars with the number of these organisms, which give no warning because their toxins are odorless, tasteless and invisible to the naked eye.

Pack Wise to Stay Safe

- Use hot soapy water on hands, countertops, utensils and cutting boards before and after food preparation.

- Keep cold foods cold (below 60 degrees) and hot foods hot (above 125 degrees).

Use thermal containers. Give them a headstart by chilling cold containers with ice water or a short freezer visit, and preheating hot containers with boiling water. Make sure the hot food is almost boiling hot when going into the thermos.

- Freeze your juice box, water or beverage in a plastic container; it will serve as a cold pack to help keep your foods cool.

If your work site has no refrigerator to store your lunch, you might want to invest in a mini-cooler or an insulated bag with a freezer-pack or frozen beverage. With such care, many sandwiches will stay safe and fresh until lunchtime. If you are taking frozen leftovers, don't remove them from the freezer until you get up in the morning—they will thaw, yet stay cold until lunch.

Use the recipes on the following pages to prepare delicious midday meals—whether you are lunching at home or on the run! Then find a quiet spot and enjoy a time of refreshing—body and spirit. With a little creativity and planning, this time can become a welcomed respite to your busy day.

Sensational Sides

To round out your lunchbox thermos, you may want to add one of these sensational sides to provide the needed simple carbohydrate or protein.

- Whole or cut fruit
- Black Bean and Corn Salsa (pg. 99)
- Raw veggies and dip
- Mango Salsa (pg. 130)
- Gazpacho (pg. 99)
- Mixed Green Salad with dressing on the side (pg. 109)
- Sliced cucumber salad

Lunch in a Thermos

lunches & soups
TWENTY-TWO MEALS

A Cold One

Fill a wide-mouthed thermos with ice water for a few minutes; pour out the water and fill with your very cold lunch creation. This will keep it chilled until lunch.

- Chicken and Pasta Salad (pg. 85)
- Roasted Red Pepper and Tortellini Salad (pg. 87)
- Tuscan Bean Salad (pg. 87)
- Confetti Chicken Salad (pg. 94)
- Gazpacho (pg. 99)
- Cottage cheese and fruit
- Fresh fruit shake

A Hot One

Fill a wide-mouthed thermos with very hot water for a few minutes; pour out the water and fill with almost boiling food that will be ready for your steaming hot lunch.

- Chili in a Hurry (pg. 102)
- Red Lentil Chili (pg. 103)
- Pasta e Fagioli (pg. 101)
- Smoked Turkey and White Bean Soup (pg. 100)
- Leftover lasagna, spaghetti or any pasta dish
- Macaroni and cheese
- Beef Stew (pg. 127)
- Leftover Risotto (pg. 109)
- Black beans and rice

The Lunchbox Package

Wrapping

- Whole-wheat, rye or pumpernickel bread
- Whole-grain kaiser or hamburger buns
- Whole-wheat English muffins
- Low-fat flour tortilla (preferably whole wheat)
- Whole-wheat bagels
- Whole-wheat pita bread
- Crepes
- Lettuce leaves
- Focaccia bread

Contents

- Lean, sliced meats (turkey, chicken breast, roast beef, Canadian bacon, low-fat ham)
- Nonfat or low-fat cheese
- Bean spreads
- Tuna or salmon
- Boiled egg whites or tofu
- Peanut butter and fruit
- Cottage cheese with trail mix

Trimmings

- Romaine or leaf lettuce
- Sliced vegetables (peppers, tomato, cucumbers)
- Spice sprouts
- Shredded carrots
- Mustard or light mayonnaise
- Salsa
- Sensational spreads (pg. 60)

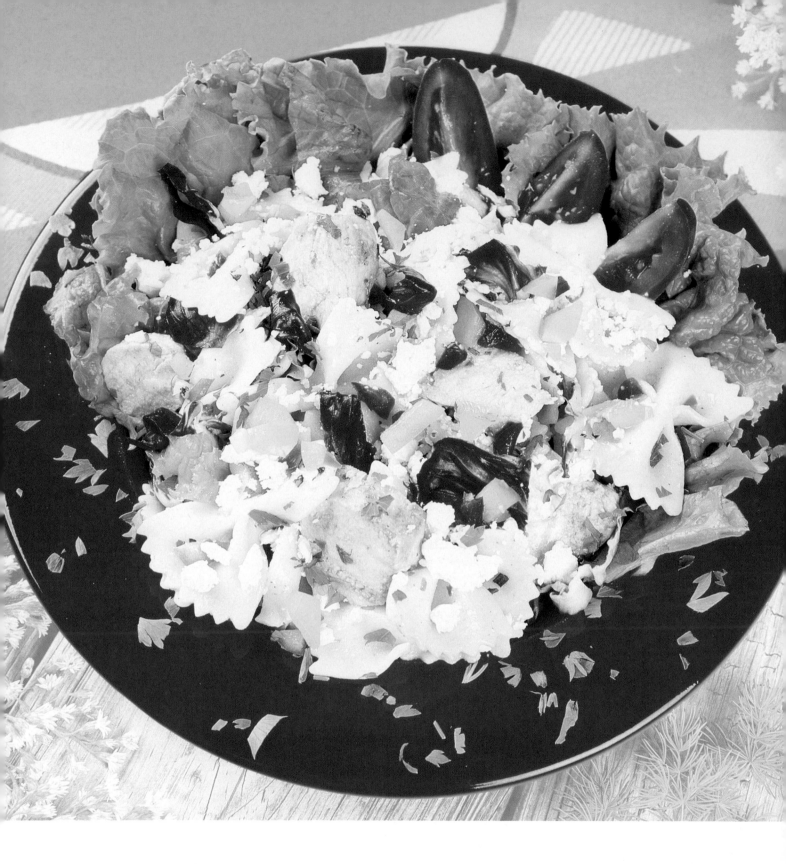

The exciting flavors of Greek salad: Feta, pepperoncinis and a fabulous Greek dressing all bring a taste sensation to this luncheon salad that could easily become a quick and elegant meal. The pasta salad can be made and kept refrigerated for up to five days; the smoked chicken—or shrimp, scallops or turkey, if you prefer—can be added at serving time.

Greek Pasta Salad

turkey, feta cheese (protein)
pasta (complex carb.)
vegetables (simple carb.)

Greek Pasta

4 cups bowtie pasta, cooked and
   cooled
1 red bell pepper, finely diced
1 green bell pepper, finely diced
1 yellow pepper, finely diced
½ red onion, finely minced
2 Tbsp. chopped fresh herbs (cilantro,
   basil, rosemary, thyme)
1 cup Greek Vinaigrette
1 tsp. creole seasoning

Combine all ingredients. Allow to marinate at least one hour.
Makes 4 servings.

Per Serving: 204 Calories

Protein 7 gr.   Carb. 35 gr.
Fat 4 gr.   Cal. from fat 18%
Chol. 0 mg.   Sodium 420 mg.

Greek Vinaigrette

¼ cup olive oil
1¼ cups rice wine vinegar
¾ cup chicken stock (fat-free/low salt)
¼ cup Dijon mustard
½ cup pepperoncini juice
1 Tbsp. minced garlic
1 Tbsp. minced shallots
1 tsp. creole seasoning
2 Tbsp. chopped fresh herbs (cilantro,
   basil, rosemary, thyme)
1 Tbsp. chopped fresh oregano
   (or 1 tsp. dried)

In a large bowl, whisk together ingredients. Refrigerate.
Makes 24 servings, 2 Tbsp. each.

Per Serving: 21 Calories

Protein 0 gr.   Carb. 1 gr.
Fat 2 gr.   Cal. from fat 66%
Chol. 0 mg.   Sodium 139 mg.

Chicken and Pasta Salad

12 oz. smoked (or roasted) chicken
   breast
1 recipe of Greek Pasta
2 cups fresh spinach, washed, stemmed
   and snipped
2 cups romaine or red leaf lettuce
1 cup radicchio leaves,* torn
4 plum tomatoes, quartered
½ cup feta cheese, crumbled
¼ cup Greek Vinaigrette
2 Tbsp. chopped fresh herbs (cilantro,
   basil, rosemary, thyme)

*   may use extra lettuce instead

Cut chicken breast into chunks; mix with Greek Pasta. Place spinach, romaine and radicchio on each of four plates; top with pasta salad. Add tomatoes and crumbled feta cheese. Ladle 1 Tbsp. of Greek Vinaigrette onto each plate, then sprinkle with herbs.
Serves 4.

Per Serving: 357 Calories

Protein 28 gr.   Carb. 41 gr.
Fat 9 gr.   Cal. from fat 22%
Chol. 0 mg.   Sodium 720 mg.

Viva La Vinaigrettes

The best vinaigrettes are made from the most flavorful vinegars, such as balsamic and rice wine vinegar, and are infused with herbs, such as basil, dill, rosemary or tarragon. Those made with fruit, blueberries, cranberries or raspberries are wonderful as well.

Make a lower-fat vinaigrette by replacing half of the oil with defatted chicken stock, vegetable or tomato juice, or fruit juices such as mango or pineapple. You may thicken the dressing by blending it with ½ tsp. cornstarch, ¼ cup cooked rice or 1 to 2 chunks cooked potato.

Chicken Quesadillas

chicken, cheese (protein)
tortilla (complex carb.)
vegetables (simple carb.)

Salsa Pizzazz

Salsa is a highly seasoned sauce, used either for dipping, topping or as a garnish. Originally made with a base of chopped tomatoes, today's salsas can be made with almost anything, even fruit.

Use warm salsa as a perfect topping for grilled meats or fish, or add 2 to 3 tablespoons salsa to cooked vegetables or salad to give pizzazz—and flavor. Spoon salsa atop baked potatoes or toss some in with hash browns. Use it as sauce for meatloaf to update an old-fashioned favorite. Salsa never lets you down!

Chicken Quesadillas

1 medium onion, sliced
½ large green bell pepper, diced
½ large red bell pepper, diced
2 Tbsp. chicken stock (fat-free/low salt)
1 tsp. minced garlic
8 large mushrooms, cleaned and sliced
⅛ tsp. cumin
⅛ tsp. crushed red pepper
pinch cayenne pepper
2 Tbsp. rice wine vinegar
1 tsp. chopped fresh cilantro
1 lb. boneless, skinless chicken breast
1 tsp. Mrs. Dash seasoning
1 tsp. creole seasoning
6 burrito-sized, fat-free flour tortillas
¾ cup grated part-skim cheddar cheese
1 cup mixed lettuces
2 cups Black Bean and Corn Salsa (pg. 55)
3 Tbsp. nonfat sour cream
½ cup Spicy Tomato Salsa

Spray a nonstick skillet with cooking spray and heat. Add onion, peppers and chicken stock and quickly sauté. Add garlic, mushrooms, cumin, crushed red pepper and cayenne pepper. Cook for 2 minutes, stirring frequently. Add vinegar and cilantro, and cook until most of the liquid evaporates, about 2 minutes.

Sprinkle chicken breasts with seasonings and grill. Cut crosswise into ½-inch strips.

Lay each tortilla on surface of another hot nonstick skillet or griddle. Put 2 Tbsp. vegetable mixture, 2 oz. chicken (½ cup) and 2 Tbsp. cheese on one-half of each tortilla. Fold over, and grill until browned and crispy and cheese is melted.

Cut each quesadilla into 3 triangles and lay on plate next to lettuce. Top lettuce with ⅓ cup

Black Bean and Corn Salsa. Serve with ¼ cup salsa topped with ½ Tbsp. nonfat sour cream.

Makes 6 servings, 3 triangles per serving.

Per Serving: 431 Calories

Protein 42 gr.	Carb. 50 gr.
Fat 7 gr.	Cal. from fat 15%
Chol. 84 mg.	Sodium 599 mg.

Spicy Tomato Salsa

1½ lbs. plum tomatoes, seeded and diced
½ cup finely diced red onion
1 jalapeño, stemmed, seeded and finely diced
1 Tbsp. chopped fresh cilantro
1 tsp. cumin
1 tsp. creole seasoning
¼ tsp. cracked black pepper
2 cloves garlic, minced
juice of 1 lime

Combine all ingredients in a medium-sized bowl. Refrigerate to allow flavors to blend.
Use 2 Tbsp. per serving.

Per Serving: 15 Calories

Protein 0 gr.	Carb. 3 gr.
Fat 0 gr.	Cal. from fat 0%
Chol. 0 mg.	Sodium 160 mg.

Terrific Lunchtime Salads

Tuscan Bean Salad

beans, chickpeas (protein)
peppers, peas (complex carb.)
mixed greens (simple carb.)

1 cup cooked black beans, drained
1 cup cooked dark red kidney beans, drained
1 cup cooked chickpeas, drained
2 cloves garlic, minced
2 tsp. minced shallots
8 pieces jarred roasted red peppers, slivered
3 plum tomatoes, quartered
⅓ cup sliced banana peppers
½ cup white wine*
1½ cups rice wine vinegar
2 cups chicken stock (fat-free/low salt)
2 tsp. arrowroot (or 1 Tbsp. cornstarch)
2 tsp. Mrs. Dash seasoning
1 tsp. creole seasoning
5 Tbsp. chopped fresh herbs (cilantro, basil, rosemary, thyme), divided
1 bag (12 oz.) baby mixed greens or 3 cups torn lettuce
2 cups spinach or red leaf lettuce
½ cup Greek Vinaigrette (pg. 51)
1 cup frozen green peas, thawed

* or substitute dealcoholized wine or more chicken stock

Combine beans, chickpeas, garlic, shallots, red pepper, tomatoes and banana peppers.

In separate bowl, combine white wine, vinegar, chicken stock, arrowroot, seasonings and 3 Tbsp. chopped herbs. Pour over bean mixture, toss gently, then marinate at least 4 hours.

To serve, toss with mixed greens, spinach and Greek Vinaigrette. Add green peas. Sprinkle with remaining chopped herbs.

Serves 4.

Per Serving: 291 Calories

Protein 16 gr.	Carb. 51 gr.
Fat 4 gr.	Cal. from fat 12%
Chol. 0 mg.	Sodium 502 mg.

Roasted Red Pepper and Tortellini Salad

cheese (protein)
pasta (complex carb.)
melon (simple carb.)

10 oz. light cheese tortellini (purchase in grocery refrigerated sections)
1 jar (7½ oz.) roasted red peppers, drained and sliced
¼ cup chopped fresh basil or parsley
3 Tbsp. capers, rinsed
2 scallions, trimmed, finely chopped
2 cloves garlic, minced
½ cup feta cheese, crumbled
¼ cup Balsamic Marinade (pg. 56)
¼ tsp. creole seasoning

_____

• Serve with ¼ cantaloupe, sliced, per serving.

In a large saucepan of boiling water, cook tortellini al dente, 4 to 6 minutes. Drain in a colander and rinse well with cold water.

Transfer to a large bowl; add remaining ingredients.

Serves 4.

Per Serving: 313 Calories

Protein 19 gr.	Carb. 39 gr.
Fat 9 gr.	Cal. from fat 25%
Chol. 41 mg.	Sodium 763 mg.

lunches & soups

TWENTY-TWO MEALS

Eat Your Veggies!

Your mother sure was right when she told you to "eat your veggies!" Here's why: Recent studies show vegetables to be full of nutrients that are champion fighters against disease— including both cancer and heart disease. And the best way to get these super-nutrients is from real foods—not supplements.

Go for bright, vivid colors when shopping for fruits and vegetables—it's a sure sign that they are loaded with protection.

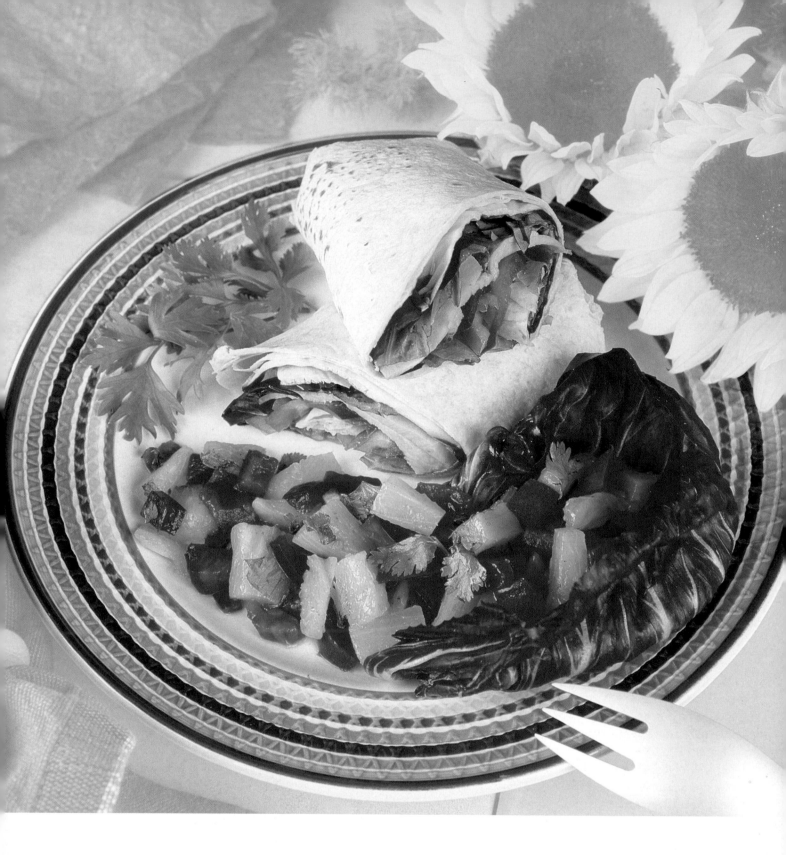

This sandwich will rewrite your definition of the lunchtime sandwich—and give you an entirely new perspective on tortillas! They aren't just for burritos any longer—they serve as a terrific wrapper for any sandwich filling. Serve with another taste sensation, Pineapple Tomato Salsa, and you'll be ready for a fiesta—not a siesta—after this lunch.

Summer Fiesta Lunch

turkey, beans (protein)
tortilla (complex carb.)
pineapple, tomato (simple carb.)

Turkey Tortilla Roll

2 Tbsp. Black Bean Dip*
2 Tbsp. fat-free sour cream
1 burrito-sized fat-free flour tortilla
1 cup shredded mixed lettuces
2 oz. turkey breast, sliced
4 strips red bell peppers
4 strips green bell peppers
2 tomato slices

* may use purchased dip or make
Black Bean Dip

• Serve with ⅓ cup Pineapple
Tomato Salsa.

Spread Black Bean Dip and fat-free sour cream onto tortilla to cover. Top with lettuce, turkey, peppers and tomatoes.

Roll tortilla tightly burrito style, secure with toothpicks and cut in half.

Serves 1.

Per Serving: 262 Calories

Protein 24 gr.   Carb. 37 gr.
Fat 2 gr.   Cal. from fat 7%
Chol. 40 mg.   Sodium 433 mg.

Pineapple Tomato Salsa

1 pineapple, diced
1 red bell pepper, cut into strips
2 plum tomatoes, diced
juice of 1 lime
1 Tbsp. chopped fresh cilantro
¼ tsp. dried coriander seed
1 tsp. creole seasoning
1 radicchio or red cabbage leaf

Mix all ingredients together except radicchio. Refrigerate at least 1 hour to blend flavors. Spoon Pineapple Tomato Salsa onto radicchio leaf placed on plate.

This salsa will keep in the refrigerator for 4 to 5 days.

Makes 4 servings, ⅓ cup each.

Per Serving: 32 Calories

Protein 0 gr.   Carb. 8 gr.
Fat 0 gr.   Cal. from fat 0%
Chol. 0 mg.   Sodium 268 mg.

Black Bean Dip

2 cans (15 oz. each) black beans, drained
  and rinsed
4 Tbsp. finely chopped canned or fresh
  jalapeño peppers
2 Tbsp. red wine vinegar
2 tsp. chili powder (or to taste)
½ tsp. creole seasoning
¼ tsp. cumin
1 Tbsp. minced onion
1 tsp. minced garlic
1 Tbsp. chopped fresh parsley

Place the beans, pepper, vinegar, chili powder, creole seasoning and cumin in a blender. Blend the ingredients until they are smooth. Transfer the mixture to a bowl.

Stir in the onion, garlic and parsley, and serve. Makes 12 servings, ⅓ cup per serving.

Per Serving: 117 Calories

Protein 8 gr.   Carb. 21 gr.
Fat 0 gr.   Cal. from fat 0%
Chol. 0 mg.   Sodium 68 mg.

Fat-Free Sour Cream

Fat-free sour cream is a wonderful substitute for regular sour cream. It's made from skim milk instead of cream, so you avoid the fat naturally without adding extra chemicals or sugars.

(Fat-free mayonnaise, on the other hand, is manufactured by adding the chemicals and sugars, so I recommend light mayonnaise instead.)

lunches & soups

TWENTY-TWO MEALS

Choose Great Greens

Leave iceberg lettuce at the store. Instead, come home with the greenest lettuces you can find. Besides romaine, green and red leaf, spinach and watercress, try arugula, Belgian endive, curly endive, frizee, escarole, dandelion greens, mache, mustard greens and radicchio.

Look for greens that are crisp and free of blemishes. Wash and dry, then store by wrapping in dry paper towels in a tightly sealed plastic bag. One pound of greens yields about 6 cups of torn lettuce.

Super Sandwiches

Mango-Chicken Salad Sandwiches

chicken (protein)
English muffin (complex carb.)
mango (simple carb.)

1 ½ Tbsp. light mayonnaise
1 Tbsp. minced celery
1 Tbsp. chopped fresh cilantro or parsley
2 tsp. fresh lemon juice
1 Tbsp. chopped red bell pepper
½ tsp. creole seasoning
⅔ cup peeled and diced mango
1 can (6 oz.) of water-packed chicken, drained*
2 green or red leaf lettuce leaves
2 whole-wheat English muffins, split and toasted
1 Tbsp. slivered almonds, toasted

* *you may substitute fresh crabmeat or water-packed solid white tuna*

Combine the first 6 ingredients in a bowl; stir well. Add mango and chicken; toss gently to coat.

Arrange 1 lettuce leaf on each muffin half, top with ¾ cup chicken mixture and sprinkle with almonds. Place on plate, laying top half of muffin against sandwich.

Serves 2.

Per Serving: 408 Calories

Protein 30 gr.	Carb. 51 gr.
Fat 9 gr.	Cal. from fat 20%
Chol. 70 mg.	Sodium 744 mg.

Grilled Vegetable Baguettes

beans (protein)
French bread (complex carb.)
vegetables (simple carb.)

1 eggplant, cut lengthwise into ¼-inch slices
1 zucchini, cut lengthwise into ¼-inch slices
1 yellow squash, cut lengthwise into ¼-inch slices
1 red bell pepper, sliced thin
1 cup Balsamic Marinade (pg. 56)
1 (1 lb.) baguette (a long, thin loaf of French bread)
2 cups Bean and Garlic Pesto (pg. 60)
1 red onion, sliced thin
1 tomato, sliced thin
1 cup loosely packed spinach, washed and stemmed

● **Serve with mixed greens or Chilled Cucumber Salad (pg. 116).**

Marinate sliced eggplant, zucchini, squash and red pepper in Balsamic Marinade for at least 1 hour.

Grill or broil eggplant, zucchini, squash and red pepper until crisp tender.

Cut baguette in half lengthwise. Spread cut side of each half with pesto. On bottom half of baguette, layer eggplant, zucchini, squash, red pepper, onion, tomato and spinach. Top with remaining half of baguette and cut into 6 pieces.

Serves 6.

Per Serving: 316 Calories

Protein 13 gr.	Carb. 55 gr.
Fat 5.5 gr.	Cal. from fat 15%
Chol. 0 mg.	Sodium 470 mg.

Dilled Tortilla Roll

cheese (protein)
tortilla (complex carb.)
cantaloupe (simple carb.)

Dilled Tortilla Roll

¼ cup fat-free cream cheese
1 tsp. chopped fresh dill
1 tsp. chopped fresh herbs (cilantro, basil, rosemary, thyme)
¼ tsp. Mrs. Dash Garlic and Herb Seasoning
⅛ tsp. cracked black pepper
2 tsp. lemon juice
1 burrito-sized, fat-free flour tortilla
2 radicchio leaves
⅓ cup shredded lettuce
2 Tbsp. diced, seeded cucumber
½ small tomato, diced

- Serve with ¼ cup Cucumber Dill Dressing for dipping and ¼ cantaloupe.

Mix light cream cheese with dill, herbs, seasoning, pepper and lemon juice.

Spread cheese mixture on flour tortilla; top with radicchio leaves and sprinkle with lettuce, cucumber and tomato. Roll tortilla burrito style and fasten with 2 toothpicks. Cut in half.
Serves 1.

Per Serving: 222 Calories

Protein 12.5 gr.	Carb. 34 gr.
Fat 4 gr.	Cal. from fat 16%
Chol. 30 mg.	Sodium 357 mg.

Cucumber Dill Dressing

6 oz. light cream cheese
⅓ cup farmer's cheese
1 cup skim milk
1 large cucumber, peeled, seeded and chopped
1½ Tbsp. Dijon mustard
2 cloves garlic, minced
¼ tsp. cracked black pepper
1 tsp. creole seasoning
1 Tbsp. olive oil
juice of 1 lemon
½ tsp. Tabasco
2 Tbsp. chopped fresh dill

Blend cheeses together with skim milk. Add other ingredients, except dill, and blend until smooth. Stir in dill.
Makes 24 servings, ¼ cup each.

Per Serving: 38 Calories

Protein 1.5 gr.	Carb. 1 gr.
Fat 3 gr.	Cal. from fat 71%
Chol. 3 mg.	Sodium 34 mg.

Tortilla Tips

Flour tortillas are for more than just Mexican food—they are the perfect sandwich wrapper for a variety of fillings. They make terrific pizza crusts and can bake into crispy additions to desserts (pg. 164).

Find tortillas in the refrigerated section of supermarkets, and look for the low-fat and fat-free versions (made without lard). You can also get the whole-wheat variety—they are full-flavored and nutritious.

To warm tortillas, wrap them loosely in paper towels or wax paper and pop into the microwave on high for 15 seconds per two tortillas.

lunches & soups

Make Your Own Cheese Blends

Because fat-free cheeses do not melt as quickly or as easily as traditional high-fat cheeses, make your own cheese blends and keep handy. These are two of my favorite blends: a part-skim mozzarella/Parmesan blend, consisting of 3 parts grated part-skim mozzarella and 1 part grated Parmesan; and a blend of part-skim mozzarella with part-skim sharp cheddar cheese, consisting of 3 parts part-skim mozzarella and 1 part cheddar.

You can pay the price to buy cheese pre-grated, or grate it ahead of time and refrigerate in a plastic bag until ready to use. Four ounces of block cheese will yield one cup grated.

Pizza Pizzazz

Vegetable Tortilla Pizza

cheese (protein)
tortilla (complex carb.)
vegetables (simple carb.)

2 fajita-sized, fat-free flour tortillas
⅓ cup fat-free mozzarella/Parmesan cheese blend, divided (left column)
¼ cup Tomato Basil Sauce (pg. 59)
1 Tbsp. chopped fresh herbs (cilantro, basil, rosemary, thyme), divided
6 strips red bell pepper
6 strips green bell pepper
6 strips yellow bell pepper
3 broccoli florets
¼ small red onion, diced

Preheat oven to 450 degrees.

Lay one tortilla on round wire mesh pan. Sprinkle it with 2 Tbsp. cheese blend; top with remaining tortilla.

Brush the top of tortilla with Tomato Basil Sauce and sprinkle with ½ Tbsp. herbs. Lay peppers, broccoli and onions on top of sauce. Sprinkle with the remaining cheese blend.

Bake until lightly browned and crisp, about 5 minutes. Sprinkle with remaining herbs.

Serves 1.

Per Serving: 309 Calories

Protein 18 gr.	Carb. 48 gr.
Fat 5 gr.	Cal. from fat 14%
Chol. 24 mg.	Sodium 460 mg.

English Muffin Pizzas

cheese (protein)
English muffin (complex carb.)
eggplant, tomato (simple carb.)

2 egg whites
½ cup seasoned dry bread crumbs (purchased)
1 large eggplant, sliced thin
2 tsp. olive oil
4 English muffins, split
1½ cups Tomato Basil Sauce (pg. 59)
1 tomato, sliced thin
2 cups part-skim mozzarella/Parmesan cheese blend (right column)
½ tsp. dried basil
½ tsp. creole seasoning

Preheat oven to 350 degrees.

Lightly beat egg whites in a pie plate. Place bread crumbs on a piece of wax paper. Dip eggplant into egg whites, then into bread crumbs.

Spray a nonstick skillet with cooking spray. Add olive oil and warm it over medium-high heat. Add eggplant slices and cook until golden, 2 to 3 minutes on each side.

Place muffin halves on a baking sheet. Spread each with 3 Tbsp. of Tomato Basil Sauce. Place ¼ of the eggplant and tomato slices on each muffin half. Sprinkle each with cheese, basil and seasoning. Bake until cheese melts, 15 to 20 minutes.

Serves 4.

Per Serving: 377 Calories

Protein 21 gr.	Carb. 54 gr.
Fat 8.5 gr.	Cal. from fat 20%
Chol. 24 mg.	Sodium 622 mg.

Pizza or Nachos, Anyone?

Spinach and Mushroom Pita Pizza

cheese (protein)
pita (complex carb.)
vegetables (simple carb.)

1 oz. (or ½ cup dried) assorted mushrooms
4 dried shiitake mushrooms
2 cloves garlic, chopped
1 cup fresh spinach, washed and
  stemmed
½ tsp. creole seasoning
1 tsp. Mrs. Dash seasoning
2 whole-wheat pita breads
¼ cup Tomato Basil Sauce (pg. 59)
2 plum tomatoes, peeled, seeded and
  quartered
½ cup feta cheese, crumbled

Preheat oven to 475 degrees.
Soak the dried mushrooms in cold water until
hydrated; squeeze dry. Spray a nonstick skillet
with cooking spray and sauté mushrooms, shii-
takes and garlic until tender. Add spinach and
seasonings. Cover and allow to steam for
approximately 1 minute until spinach wilts.
Spray both pitas lightly with cooking spray.
Brush with Tomato Basil Sauce. Cover with
spinach-mushroom mixture, leaving a ¾-inch
border. Top with tomato quarters and cheese.
Bake until warmed and crispy, 5 minutes.
Serves 2.

Per Serving: 234 Calories

Protein 11 gr.	Carb. 33 gr.
Fat 7 gr.	Cal. from fat 25%
Chol. 25 mg.	Sodium 755 mg.

Guiltless Nachos

cheese, beans (protein)
chips (complex carb.)
salsa, vegetables (simple carb.)

3 oz. baked tortilla chips (about ¼ bag)
½ cup Black Bean Dip (pg. 61), warmed
¼ cup nonfat sour cream
½ small tomato, chopped
¾ cup grated part-skim mozzarella
¼ cup grated part-skim sharp cheddar
¼ cup spicy salsa (purchased)
1 Tbsp. green onion, sliced thin
2 Tbsp. finely chopped red, green and
  yellow bell pepper

Lay half of chips onto large oval platter.
Spoon half of bean dip and 2 Tbsp. of fat-free
sour cream onto chips. Top with remaining
chips, then remaining bean dip. Sprinkle with
chopped tomato.
Mix together mozzarella and cheddar
cheeses; sprinkle onto chips. Place under
broiler just until cheese is melted. Spoon on
salsa and dot with remaining sour cream.
Sprinkle with green onions and confetti mix
of finely chopped peppers.
Serves 2. Can also serve as a whole platter
for an appetizer munchie.

Per Serving: 259 Calories

Protein 21 gr.	Carb. 36 gr.
Fat 4 gr.	Cal. from fat 14%
Chol. 11 mg.	Sodium 724 mg.

lunches & soups

TWENTY-TWO MEALS

Baked Pita Chips

*Pita has unlimited pos-
sibilities—it can be
used as a sandwich
pouch, a quick pizza
crust or baked to make
terrific dipping chips.*

*Make pita chips by sep-
arating pita rounds hori-
zontally. Spray the
rounds with cooking
spray and lightly
season to taste with salt
and pepper. Stack the
rounds, then cut the
stack into 12 wedges.
Arrange in a single
layer on a
nonstick baking sheet
and bake at 350
degrees for 8 minutes
or until golden brown.
Cool on paper towels
and store in an
airtight container.*

Confetti Chicken Salad

chicken (protein)
corn (complex carb.)
tomatoes, peppers (simple carb.)

Confetti Chicken Salad

12 oz. boneless, skinless chicken breasts
2 cups chicken broth (fat-free/low salt)
1 recipe Cumin-Dijon Dressing
3 ears of corn, cooked and cooled
24 cherry tomatoes, halved
6 radishes, sliced thin
½ red bell pepper, sliced
4 cups romaine leaves, torn into bite-sized pieces

- Serve with 4 oranges, peeled and sliced.

In a skillet over medium heat, bring chicken and broth to a boil. Reduce heat to medium low. Cover and poach chicken until it is no longer pink, 6 to 8 minutes. Transfer chicken to cutting board and cut into bite-sized pieces. Add Cumin-Dijon Dressing to chicken and toss to coat.

Cut kernels from corn cobs. Add corn, tomatoes, radishes and peppers to chicken. Toss until well combined. Arrange lettuce on a platter and top with the salad. Surround each salad with 1 orange, sliced.

Serves 4.

Per Serving: 312 Calories

Protein 22 gr.	Carb. 38 gr.
Fat 8 gr.	Cal. from fat 23%
Chol. 48 mg.	Sodium 220 mg.

Cumin-Dijon Dressing

3 Tbsp. lemon juice
1 Tbsp. olive oil
2 Tbsp. chicken stock (fat-free/low salt)
1 Tbsp. red wine vinegar
1 tsp. cumin
1 tsp. Dijon mustard
2 cloves garlic, minced
½ tsp. creole seasoning

Whisk lemon juice, oil, chicken stock, vinegar, cumin, mustard, garlic and seasoning in a bowl. Set aside to use with Confetti Chicken Salad.

This dressing may also be used with other salads and is a delicious addition to chicken or turkey sandwiches.

Makes 4 servings, 2 Tbsp. each.

Per Serving: 31 Calories

Protein 0 gr.	Carb. 0 gr.
Fat 3.4 gr.	Cal. from fat 98%
Chol. 0 mg.	Sodium 150 mg.

Removing Corn From the Cob

To remove corn from its cob, begin by cutting a small piece off the tip to make it flat. Holding the stem edge, stand the cob upright with the flat end on a plate. Use a firm-bladed, very sharp knife to cut downward, removing the corn 3 or 4 rows at a time. To get the "milk" of the corn, use the back of the blade to scrape what's left of the juice from the cobs.

Soup and Sandwich Combo

turkey, cheese (protein)
bread (complex carb.)
gazpacho (simple carb.)

Market Club Sandwich

3 thin slices marble rye bread
½ Tbsp. light mayonnaise
2 tsp. Dijon mustard
2 green lettuce leaves
2 oz. smoked turkey breast, sliced thin
1 oz. Jarlsberg Lite Swiss cheese
2 slices tomato
1 radicchio leaf

Spread bread with mayo and mustard. Top one slice of bread with one lettuce leaf and 1 oz. turkey, then add second slice of bread. Top with another lettuce leaf, Swiss cheese, tomato slice, radicchio leaf and turkey. Top with remaining slice of bread.
Serves 1.

Per Serving: 355 Calories

Protein 29 gr.	Carb. 38 gr.
Fat 9 gr.	Cal. from fat 24%
Chol. 59 mg.	Sodium 706 mg.

Gazpacho

1 medium red bell pepper, seeded and finely diced
1 medium green bell pepper, seeded and finely diced
½ cucumber (European is best) peeled, seeded and finely diced
½ small red onion, finely diced
2 tomatoes, finely diced
1½ cups (12 oz.) V-8 juice
1½ cups (12 oz.) tomato juice
1 Tbsp. white wine vinegar
1 clove garlic, minced
1 tsp. Tabasco
¼ cup chopped fresh basil
¼ tsp. cumin
1 tsp. creole seasoning

Combine ingredients. Chill. Serve cold. Makes 12 small servings, ½ cup each.

Per Serving: 22 Calories

Protein 1 gr.	Carb. 5 gr.
Fat 0 gr.	Cal. from fat 0%
Chol. 0 mg.	Sodium 312 mg.

A Word About Soups

Soups make an elegant and exciting first course for any meal you want to make special. Choose one that will complement the flavors of the other dishes in the meal. For example, this zesty, chilled gazpacho is the perfect prelude to this summertime sandwich.

You can shave off a lot of preparation time by using your food processor; it chops and slices vegetables in a fraction of the time it would take to do by hand. Always start with the least moist and messy vegetable. Mushrooms, for example, should be cut and set aside before you chop something moist like peppers or tomatoes. Don't worry about wiping out the bowl between veggies—it's all going into the same pot anyway!

Grilled Turkey Burger

turkey (protein)
bun (complex carb.)
tomato, pineapple (simple carb.)

Grilled Turkey Burger

1 Turkey Burger Patty
1 multigrain hamburger bun
½ Tbsp. Garlic Aioli
1 large lettuce leaf
2 slices tomato
2 red onion rings

- Serve with ⅓ cup Pineapple
  Tomato Salsa (pg. 55) in a red
  cabbage leaf.

Grill Turkey Burger Patty. Place patty on multigrain bun spread with aioli, lettuce, tomato
slices and onion.
Serves 1.

Per Serving: 403 Calories

Protein 41 gr.   Carb. 44 gr.
Fat 7 gr.   Cal. from fat 16%
Chol. 96 mg.   Sodium 724 mg.

Turkey Burger Patty

3 lbs. ground turkey breast
8 oz. Simply Potatoes hash browns,
   cooked
⅓ cup chopped fresh parsley
1 Tbsp. Mrs. Dash seasoning
½ tsp. black pepper
½ cup diced white onions
1 Tbsp. chicken stock (fat-free/low salt)
1 egg white, lightly beaten

Mix all ingredients together in food processor
or blender on rough chop until ingredients are
blended. Shape into 10 patties.
Makes 10 patties, 5½ oz. each.

Per Serving: 236 Calories

Protein 36 gr.   Carb. 6 gr.
Fat 5 gr.   Cal. from fat 19%
Chol. 96 mg.   Sodium 294 mg.

Garlic Aioli

1 cup light mayonnaise
½ cup nonfat plain yogurt
½ tsp. creole seasoning
1 Tbsp. finely chopped shallots
2 tsp. chopped fresh herbs (cilantro,
   basil, rosemary, thyme)
4 cloves garlic, minced
juice of ½ lemon

Mix together all ingredients. Refrigerate.
Makes 25 servings, 1 Tbsp. each.

Per Serving: 28 Calories

Protein 0 gr.   Carb. 1 gr.
Fat 2.5 gr.   Cal. from fat 80%
Chol. 3 mg.   Sodium 25 mg.

Grilled Fish Sandwich

fish (protein)
bun, potato (complex carb.)
vegetables (simple carb.)

Grilled Fish Sandwich

16 oz. grouper or snapper
¼ cup Balsamic Marinade (pg. 56)
4 multigrain kaiser or hamburger
   buns
2 Tbsp. Garlic Aioli (pg. 96)
4 large lettuce leaves
1 red onion, sliced into rings
1 tomato, sliced
sprinkle of chopped fresh herbs
   (cilantro, basil, rosemary, thyme)

Cut fish into 4 pieces. Marinate in Balsamic Marinade for up to 1 hour. Grill over hot coals or gas grill until done.

Spread buns with aioli and top with fish, lettuce, onion and tomato slices. Sprinkle with chopped herbs.

Serves 4.

Per Serving: 251 Calories

Protein 26 gr.	Carb. 24 gr.
Fat 4 gr.	Cal. from fat 14%
Chol. 44 mg.	Sodium 305 mg.

Herbed Potato Salad

1½ lbs. red-skinned potatoes,
   scrubbed and quartered
½ tsp. salt
1 Tbsp. white wine vinegar
½ tsp. creole seasoning
2 Tbsp. light mayonnaise
1 Tbsp. Dijon mustard
¼ cup nonfat sour cream
⅓ cup chopped celery
1 red bell pepper, julienned
¼ cup chopped green onions
1 Tbsp. chopped fresh parsley
1 Tbsp. chopped fresh dill

In a medium-sized saucepan, cover potatoes with cold water and add salt. Bring to a boil, and cook over medium heat until tender, 7 to 9 minutes. Drain in colander and gently transfer to a large bowl. Toss with vinegar and seasoning. Set the potatoes aside to cool.

In a small bowl, whisk together the mayonnaise, mustard and sour cream. Add the dressing and the rest of the ingredients to the potatoes.

Serves 6.

Per Serving: 125 Calories

Protein 3 gr.	Carb. 25 gr.
Fat 1.5 gr.	Cal. from fat 12%
Chol. 2 mg.	Sodium 142 mg.

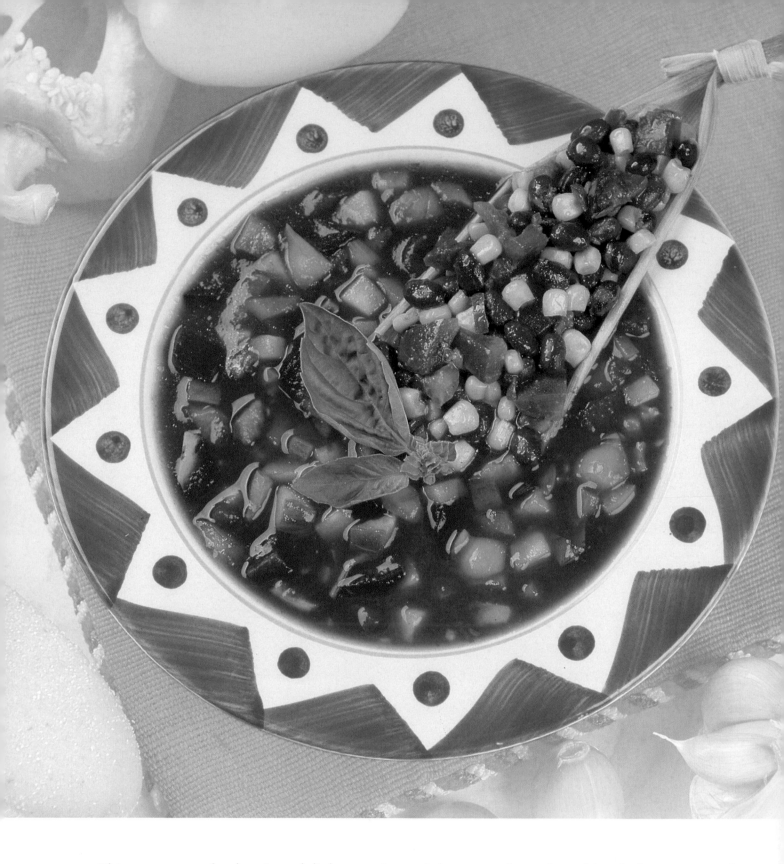

This summer refresher is a delight any time of the year. The unique blend of textures and flavors—cool yet spicy, smooth yet crispy—combined with the vivid colors provides a feast for the senses. The Black Bean and Corn Salsa is an appealing accompaniment—and a fun addition when served as pictured—in a fresh corn husk.

Gazpacho With Salsa

beans (protein)
corn (complex carb.)
tomatoes, vegetables (simple carb.)

Gazpacho*

3 medium red bell peppers, seeded and finely diced
3 medium green bell peppers, seeded and finely diced
1 European cucumber, peeled, seeded and finely diced
1 small red onion, finely diced
6 tomatoes, finely diced
1 can (40 oz.) V-8 juice
1 can (40 oz.) tomato juice
3 Tbsp. white wine vinegar
2 garlic cloves, finely chopped
1 Tbsp. Tabasco
¼ cup chopped fresh basil
½ tsp. cumin
1 Tbsp. creole seasoning

Combine all ingredients. Chill. Serve cold. Makes 12 servings, 1½ cups each.

Per Serving: 66 Calories

Protein 3 gr.   Carb. 15 gr.
Fat 0 gr.   Cal. from fat 0%
Chol. 0 mg.   Sodium 936 mg.

*   See page 95 for smaller portion recipe.

Black Bean and Corn Salsa

2 cups black beans, drained and rinsed
1 cup frozen corn kernels, thawed
2 plum tomatoes, diced
½ red onion, minced
1 serrano pepper, minced
1 Tbsp. finely chopped cilantro
1 Tbsp. olive oil
4 cloves garlic, minced
juice of 2 limes
1 Tbsp. balsamic vinegar
1 tsp. cumin
2 tsp. hot pepper sauce
1 tsp. creole seasoning

In a large bowl, combine all ingredients and mix well. Allow to marinate at least one hour. Makes 5 servings, ⅔ cup each.

Per Serving: 158 Calories

Protein 8 gr.   Carb. 26 gr.
Fat 3 gr.   Cal. from fat 17%
Chol. 0 mg.   Sodium 236 mg.

Weight-Loss Secret: Start With Soup

Have you heard that "soup is good food"? It's true, particularly for the person working toward better portion control. Research has shown that starting your meal with soup, which has a lower caloric density than most solid foods and takes a relatively long time to eat, will often result in your eating less. It gives your brain time to register fullness before it's too late. And don't forget soup is a great one-dish meal— it's one of my favorites.

lunches & soups

TWENTY-TWO MEALS

Soups for Meals

Substitute Canned Beans in Minutes

If you don't have time to cook dry beans, you can use canned beans instead. Just empty them into a colander, then rinse and drain them well to lower the salt content.

Pasta and Chickpea Soup

beans, Parmesan cheese (protein)
pasta, beans (complex carb.)
fruit salad (simple carb.)

1 tsp. olive oil
2 cloves garlic, minced
1 can (14 oz.) whole tomatoes, drained
1 Tbsp. chopped fresh rosemary
6 cups chicken stock (fat-free/low salt)
2 cans (19 oz. each) or 4 cups cooked chickpeas, drained and rinsed
6 oz. dry penne pasta
½ tsp. creole seasoning
1 tsp. Mrs. Dash seasoning
1 ½ cup grated Parmesan cheese

● Serve with ½ cup mixed cut fruit per serving.

Spray a large stockpot with cooking spray. Add olive oil and heat. Add garlic and cook, stirring, about 1 minute. Add tomatoes and rosemary; simmer for 5 minutes, crushing the tomatoes with stirring spoon. Pour in chicken stock and bring to a simmer over medium heat.

In a small bowl, mash 1 cup of the chickpeas with a fork. Stir the mashed chickpeas into the pot, along with the penne and seasonings. Simmer uncovered until the pasta is tender, 8 to 10 minutes. Stir in the remaining whole chickpeas and heat through. Sprinkle with grated Parmesan.

Makes 8 servings, 1 ½ cups each.

Per Serving: 195 Calories

Protein 9 gr.	Carb. 32 gr.
Fat 3 gr.	Cal. from fat 14%
Chol. 16 mg.	Sodium 666 mg.

Smoked Turkey and White Bean Soup

turkey, beans (protein)
beans (complex carb.)
salad, orange (simple carb.)

1 tsp. olive oil
2 cloves garlic, minced
1 can (14 oz.) whole tomatoes, drained
2 Tbsp. chopped fresh basil (or 2 tsp. dried)
6 cups chicken stock (fat-free/low salt)
2 cans (19 oz. each) or 4 cups cooked cannelini or white beans, drained and rinsed
1 lb. smoked turkey, rough chopped
½ tsp. creole seasoning
1 tsp. Mrs. Dash seasoning

● Serve with Mixed Green Salad With Oranges (pg. 109).

Spray a large stockpot with cooking spray. Add olive oil and bring to low heat. Add garlic and cook, stirring, about 1 minute. Add tomatoes and basil; simmer for 5 minutes, crushing the tomatoes with stirring spoon. Pour in chicken stock and simmer over medium heat.

Stir in cannelini beans and smoked turkey along with the seasonings. Heat through.

Makes 10 servings, 1 ½ cups each.

Per Serving: 182 Calories

Protein 19 gr.	Carb. 17 gr.
Fat 4 gr.	Cal. from fat 21%
Chol. 33 mg.	Sodium 560 mg.

Soups for Meals (continued)

Pasta e Fagioli

beans (protein)
pasta, bread (complex carb.)
vegetables (simple carb.)

½ lb. each uncooked white, black,
  kidney and pinto beans
1 large yellow onion, chopped
2 cloves garlic, minced
1 cup cabbage, shredded
2 quarts chicken stock (fat-free/low salt)
1½ lbs. plum tomatoes, peeled, seeded
  and chopped
1 can (4 oz.) tomato paste
½ cup balsamic vinegar
2 bay leaves
2 Tbsp. chopped fresh oregano
2 Tbsp. chopped fresh thyme
1 Tbsp. chopped fresh rosemary
1 tsp. cracked black pepper
1 Tbsp. creole seasoning
1 Tbsp. Mrs. Dash seasoning
6 cups cooked whole-wheat fettucine

Wash beans and soak in water overnight. Drain.

Spray large saucepan with cooking spray. Quickly sauté onion, garlic and cabbage with 2 Tbsp. of chicken stock. Add soaked, drained beans. Add remaining chicken stock and bring to boil. Reduce to simmer and stir occasionally. Add tomatoes, tomato paste, vinegar, herbs and seasonings. Simmer for 1½ hours until beans are soft. Purée 1 cup of the beans and return to pot. Remove bay leaves.

When serving, mound ½ cup cooked fettucine into each bowl. Spoon 1½ cups of soup onto pasta.

Makes 12 servings.

Per Serving: 245 Calories

Protein 15 gr.	Carb. 46 gr.
Fat less than I gr.	Cal. from fat 2%
Chol. 0 mg.	Sodium 353 mg.

Quick Dry Bean Soak Method

Did you plan to use beans but forgot the overnight soak? Then try the quick-soak method for the beans. Just cover the beans with water in a large stock pot, bring to a boil and cover. Let boil for 5 minutes, then turn off the heat and let the beans sit on the stove for 1 hour. Rinse well, then add more liquid for the final stage of cooking.

Cooking Beans

1 Cup Dried Beans	Stock or Water	Cooking Time
Black beans	4 cups	1½ hrs.
Cannelini or white beans	3 cups	1 hr.
Garbanzo beans	4 cups	2 hrs.
Great northern beans	3½ cups	2½ to 3 hrs.
Kidney beans	3 cups	1½ hrs.
Lentils	3 cups	¾ to 1 hr.
Lima beans	2 cups	1 hr.
Navy beans	3 cups	1 hr.
Pinto beans	3 cups	1 hr.
Red beans	3 cups	1½ hrs.
Split peas	3 cups	1 hr.

Wash beans and soak in water overnight. Drain and place in large, heavy pot. Cover with stock (or water) and seasonings. Bring slowly to a boil, then reduce heat and simmer, partially covered, until tender. Bean is done when it can be "squashed" in the roof of the mouth with tongue.

Hearty Chili Meals

turkey, beans (protein)
rice, beans (complex carb.)
hearts of palm (simple carb.)

Chili in a Hurry

1 tsp. olive oil
1 small red onion, chopped
1 red bell pepper, seeded and chopped
1 green bell pepper, seeded and chopped
2 cloves garlic, minced
1 jalapeño pepper, seeded and finely chopped
1 tsp. cumin
1 ½ Tbsp. chili powder
1 tsp. creole seasoning
1 lb. ground turkey breast
2 cans (28 oz. each) whole tomatoes
1 cup chicken stock (fat-free/low salt)
1 can (15 oz.) black beans, drained

• Serve with cooked brown rice, non-fat sour cream and cilantro.

Spray a large, heavy saucepan with cooking spray and heat over medium heat. Add the olive oil, onion and bell peppers; sauté until softened, about 4 to 5 minutes. Add garlic, jalapeño pepper, cumin, chili powder and seasoning; sauté about 2 minutes more.

Add cooked turkey to sautéed vegetables and mix together. Add tomatoes and break up with spoon while sautéing.

Add chicken stock; reduce heat to low and bring to a simmer, stirring. Cook for another 15 minutes; add drained black beans. Heat through.

When serving, scoop ⅓ cup cooked brown rice into a bowl and ladle 1½ cups of chili on top. Top with 1 Tbsp. nonfat sour cream and garnish with cilantro.

Makes 8 servings.

Microwaving Ground Turkey

To cook ground turkey quickly, crumble ground turkey breast into a hard plastic colander. Cover with paper towel, place colander on a plate to catch juices and microwave on high power for 3 minutes. Stir and break up meat, and microwave for another 2 minutes or until browned.

Per Serving: 255 Calories

Protein 21 gr.	Carb. 38 gr.
Fat 2 gr.	Cal. from fat 7%
Chol. 35 mg.	Sodium 485 mg.

Hearts of Palm Vinaigrette

¼ cup orange juice
1 Tbsp. Dijon mustard
2 Tbsp. white wine vinegar
1 tsp. olive oil
2 cloves garlic, minced
½ tsp. dried whole basil
½ tsp. creole seasoning
4 lettuce leaves
1 can (14.4 oz.) hearts of palm, rinsed and cut into ½-inch slices
½ small red onion, sliced and separated into rings
2 Tbsp. chopped fresh parsley

Whisk orange juice, mustard, vinegar, olive oil, garlic, basil and seasoning together in a small bowl. Set vinaigrette aside.

Place 1 lettuce leaf on each of 4 salad plates. Arrange hearts of palm and sliced onion on lettuce leaves. Sprinkle evenly with chopped parsley. Drizzle 2 Tbsp. vinaigrette over each salad.

Serves 4.

Per Serving: 33 Calories

Protein 1 gr.	Carb. 5 gr.
Fat 1 gr.	Cal. from fat 27%
Chol. 1.5 mg.	Sodium 226 mg.

Hearty Chili Meals (continued)

lentils, cheese (protein)
lentils, cornbread (complex carb.)
vegetables (simple carb.)

Red Lentil Chili

½ lb. carrots
1 small zucchini
1 small yellow squash
½ large eggplant
½ large red onion
¾ Tbsp. olive oil
12 oz. bag red or brown lentils, rinsed
2 cups chicken stock (fat-free/low salt)
1 tsp. Mrs. Dash seasoning
1 tsp. creole seasoning
2 bay leaves
½ Tbsp. oregano
½ tsp. cumin
1 tsp. chili powder
¾ tsp. cayenne
¾ tsp. nutmeg
2 cloves garlic, minced
1 jalapeño pepper, chopped
2 cans (32 oz. each) plum tomatoes

- Serve with 1 oz. baked tortilla chips and 1 Tbsp. nonfat sour cream per serving or Southwest Cornbread.

In food processor, finely chop carrots, zucchini, squash, eggplant and onion. Spray nonstick skillet with cooking spray. Add olive oil. Heat over medium high heat. Add chopped vegetables. Sauté for 5 minutes. Add lentils, chicken stock, seasonings, herbs, spices, garlic, jalapeño peppers and tomatoes. Simmer for 2 hours.
Makes 10 servings, 1 ½ cups each.

Per Serving: 134 Calories

Protein 8 gr.	Carb. 26 gr.
Fat 1 gr.	Cal. from fat 8%
Chol. 0 mg.	Sodium 406 mg.

Southwest Cornbread

2 Tbsp. canola oil
½ cup finely chopped onion
1 egg, lightly beaten
1 Tbsp. honey
1 cup skim milk
1 cup whole-wheat pastry flour
1 cup yellow cornmeal
1 Tbsp. baking powder
½ tsp. salt
1 cup fresh or frozen corn
½ cup shredded part-skim cheddar cheese

Preheat oven to 375 degrees.
Heat oil in a small skillet. Add onion and sauté for 5 to 8 minutes or until onion is soft.
Beat together egg, honey and milk; set aside.
In a separate bowl, combine flour, cornmeal, baking powder and salt. Add to liquid mixture. Add corn, shredded cheese and onions along with all excess oil. Mix well. Spread into an 8-inch square pan coated with cooking spray.
Bake for 25 to 35 minutes or until brown and firm on top. Cut into 16 pieces.
Makes 16 servings.

Per Serving: 94 Calories

Protein 5 gr.	Carb. 15 gr.
Fat 1.5 gr.	Cal. from fat 15%
Chol. 2 mg.	Sodium 231 mg.

Prepare Less With Lentils

Lentils are the "quick and easy" legume because they don't need to soak before cooking. After rinsing in a colander, put them in a large stockpot and cover with liquid (chicken stock is best). Cover and simmer till tender, usually about 45 minutes—or a little longer if you've added acidic ingredients like tomatoes and wine, unless you add them when the lentils are almost done. Drain the liquid as soon as lentils are done, or they will continue to cook.

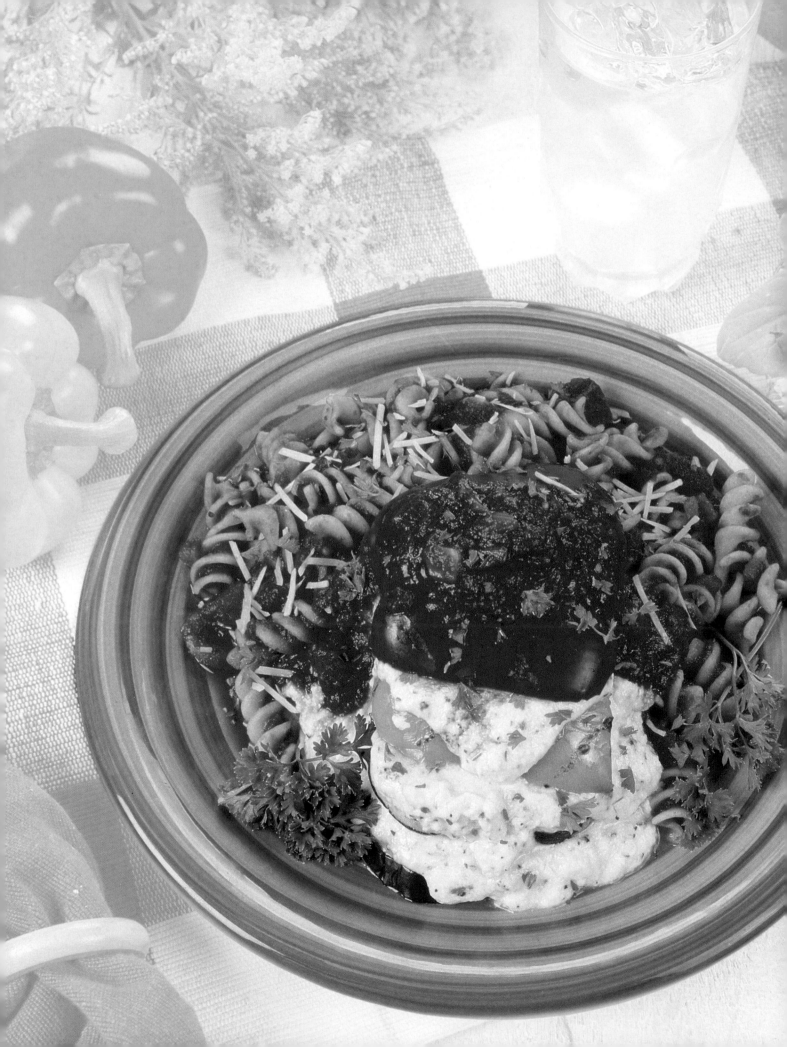

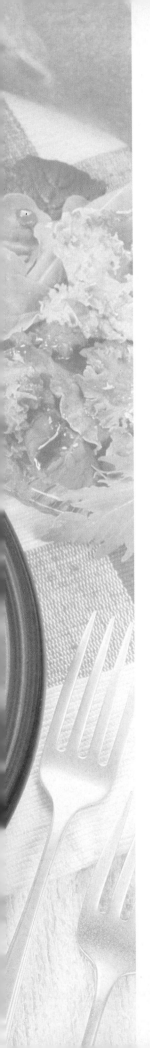

dinners
FORTY-THREE MEALS

Sitting down to a table set with a simple placemat and napkin will prepare the stage for a beautiful meal. Too often meals are eaten standing up over the sink (if eaten at all). Not only do our bodies ask, "What did you just do to me?", but our satisfaction meter asks, "Did you just inhale a meal or actually eat one?" Use these tips to enjoy dining, not just eating.

- Schedule a time for regular at-home meals.

- Sit down to the table; put on quiet, relaxing music and dine!

- Concentrate on happy and uplifting conversation or thoughts.

- Don't let the dinner table become a battleground. It should be a place of renewal, both physically and emotionally.

- Turn off the TV!

The dinner table is a great place to engage your family in conversation, which occurs far too rarely with today's busy schedules. Some super conversation starters are:

- Tell me about your day.

- What funny thing happened to you today?

- What do you think you do best?

- What's something nice that happened to you today?

- If you could trade places with anyone, who would you trade with?

- If you had three wishes, what would you wish for?

Pictured: Vegetable Lasagna (pg. 106)

- What is your favorite sport?

- If you could go anywhere in the world, where would it be?

Take an interest in the answers you hear. Give your undivided attention; listen quietly. Don't criticize, or even comment, until the answer is complete. Acknowledge the other person's feelings with words like *Oh* or *Yes* or *I see*. Really listening will keep your family close on a daily basis.

Often a sympathetic silence is all that is needed; you don't even have to say anything.

What if you're dining alone? Treat yourself just as you would others—as a special guest. And no eating over the sink allowed!

Dinner can be a magnificent transition from the stresses of the day into the relaxation of your evening. Let the food preparation be the warm-up—lots of tension can be released through chopping vegetables!

Enlist the whole family's help (and friends when they're over) in meal preparation. These occasions allow you to join together in an activity that refreshes and refuels—in all of your arenas.

Get ready—set—cook!

Vegetable Lasagna

cheeses (protein)
pasta (complex carb.)
vegetables (simple carb.)

Healthier Whole-Grain Pastas

Whole-grain pasta is more nutritious and satisfying than pasta made from refined flours; you will be full with a much smaller portion and will enjoy the hearty, nutty flavor.

Look for whole-wheat or Jerusalem artichoke pastas in your supermarket's natural food section; health food stores will also have a wide variety. Cook in a large pot, in lots of water, for about 1 minute longer than white pastas.

Try them—you'll like them!

Vegetable Lasagna

½ small eggplant, sliced very thin
1 large zucchini, sliced lengthwise
1 yellow bell pepper, quartered and flattened
1 red bell pepper, quartered and flattened
½ cup Balsamic Marinade (pg. 56)
16 oz. skim-milk ricotta cheese
1 cup feta cheese
1 Tbsp. chopped fresh oregano (or 1 tsp. dried)
1 tsp. Mrs. Dash seasoning
½ tsp. creole seasoning
2 egg whites
8 oz. dry rotini pasta (spiral), cooked
4 cups Tomato Basil Sauce, heated (pg. 59)
2 Tbsp. chopped fresh parsley

Marinate vegetables in Balsamic Marinade for at least 1 hour or up to overnight. Grill over hot coals or gas grill, or sear on both sides in hot nonstick skillet.

Mix together ricotta, feta, oregano, seasonings and egg whites until relatively smooth.

To assemble, layer individual stacks of vegetables and cheese mix on a clean counter in this order (from the bottom up):

eggplant slice
2 Tbsp. cheese mixture
zucchini slice
2 Tbsp. cheese mixture
yellow pepper quarter
2 Tbsp. cheese mixture
red bell pepper quarter

Toss pasta with 2 cups Tomato Basil Sauce. Place ½ cup of this mixture on each plate. Carefully add one of the lasagna stacks to the plate. (Use a spatula to move it.) Top both the pasta and the lasagna with ½ cup of reserved Tomato Basil Sauce, and sprinkle with chopped parsley.

Serves 4.

Per Serving: 435 Calories

Protein 34 gr.	Carb. 55 gr.
Fat 8 gr.	Cal. from fat 16%
Chol. 33 mg.	Sodium 746 mg.

Garlic Dijon Greens

8 cups mixed lettuces
2 tomatoes, quartered
1 cucumber, peeled and sliced
½ cup Roasted Garlic Dijon Vinaigrette (pg. 54)

Toss vegetables with dressing.
Serves 4.

Per Serving: 42 Calories

Protein 1 gr.	Carb. 5 gr.
Fat 2 gr.	Cal. from fat 43%
Chol. 0 mg.	Sodium 110 mg.

Eggplant Rollatini

cheeses (protein)
bread crumbs (complex carb.)
vegetables, fruit (simple carb.)

Eggplant Rollatini

1 lb. fresh spinach, washed and
    stemmed
¾ lb. eggplant, peeled and cut
    lengthwise into thin slices
½ onion, finely chopped
2 cloves garlic, minced
¼ tsp. creole seasoning
1 tsp. Mrs. Dash garlic herb seasoning
2 Tbsp. chopped fresh Italian parsley
1 Tbsp. chopped fresh basil
16 oz. skim-milk ricotta cheese
½ cup feta cheese, crumbled
1 Tbsp. grated Parmesan cheese
⅓ cup dry bread crumbs (purchased)
1 egg (or ¼ cup egg substitute)
1 egg white, slightly beaten
4 cups Tomato Basil Sauce (pg. 59)

Preheat oven to 400 degrees.

Steam spinach until wilted. Drain well and roughly chop. Reserve. Spray each side of eggplant slices with cooking spray. Bake 10 minutes, flip over and finish baking until tender. Reserve. Reduce oven temperature to 350 degrees.

Spray nonstick skillet with cooking spray. Sauté onion and garlic, adding spinach at end. Let cool. Add seasonings, herbs, cheeses and bread crumbs. Mix in egg and egg white. Chill.

To make rollatini, place 2 heaping tablespoons of spinach-cheese mixture on each eggplant slice. Roll up and place open end down in casserole dish. Cover with 1 cup Tomato Basil Sauce. Bake for 30 minutes.

Place 3 rollatini on each plate. Top with ¾ cup heated Tomato Basil Sauce.

Serves 4.

Per Serving: 309 Calories

Protein 30 gr.	Carb. 23 gr.
Fat 5 gr.	Cal. from fat 15%
Chol. 21 mg.	Sodium 785 mg.

Apple Walnut Salad

2 Tbsp. chopped walnuts
2 Tbsp. chicken stock (fat-free/low salt)
1 Tbsp. white wine vinegar
2 tsp. walnut oil (or olive oil)
1 Tbsp. finely chopped shallots
1 tsp. Dijon mustard
¼ tsp. salt
¼ tsp. cracked black pepper
8 cups washed, dried and torn mixed
    greens (red leaf, romaine, frizee,
    radicchio, arugula or bibb)
2 Granny Smith apples, cored and
    sliced thin

In a small, dry skillet over low heat, stir walnuts until lightly toasted, about 3 minutes. Transfer to a plate to cool.

In a large salad bowl, whisk together chicken stock, vinegar, oil, shallots, mustard, salt and pepper. Add greens and apples and toss thoroughly. Sprinkle with the toasted walnuts.

Per Serving: 91 Calories

Protein 2.5 gr.	Carb. 14 gr.
Fat 4 gr.	Cal. from fat 35%
Chol. 0 mg.	Sodium 159 mg.

Easy Eggplant Tips

Choose eggplants that are unspotted, firm, smooth and heavy for their size. A rounder, smoother base will mean fewer bitter seeds.

Keep eggplant refrigerated in a zip-top bag and use in five days or less. Generally, a 1-pound eggplant will yield 3 to 4 cups chopped.

Remove the bitterness from eggplant by generously salting slices on a baking sheet, covering with paper towels and weighting down with another heavy pan. Rinse and blot dry after 30 minutes.

Bowtie Pasta With Wild Mushroom Sauce

cheese (protein)
pasta (complex carb.)
vegetables (simple carb.)

Why Not Wild Mushrooms?

Wild mushrooms add a rich, exotic flavor to dishes. Look for:

- *Chanterelle (bright yellow-orange and trumpet-shaped)*

- *Enoki (long, spaghetti-like, firm stems with snow-white caps)*

- *Morel (cone-shaped, honey-combed and golden brown)*

- *Oyster (fan-shaped cap; small ones are best)*

- *Porcinis and porto-bellas (enormous large caps with a rich, beefy taste. Looks woodlike; light brown in color)*

- *Shiitake (dark brown floppy cap 8–10 inches in diameter)*

Rehydrate dried mushrooms by covering and soaking in warm water for about 30 minutes, then rinse and blot with paper towels.

Bowtie Pasta With Wild Mushroom Sauce

2 oz. dried porcini mushrooms
2 tsp. olive oil
2 cloves garlic, minced
1 red onion, sliced thin
1 red bell pepper, cut into strips
2 Tbsp. chopped fresh basil
1 tsp. dried oregano
½ tsp. creole seasoning
¾ cup fresh mushrooms, trimmed and sliced
1 can (14 oz.) plum tomatoes
1 ½ Tbsp. chopped fresh parsley
12 oz. dry bowtie pasta, cooked
½ cup grated Parmesan cheese
2 Tbsp. chopped fresh herbs (cilantro, basil, rosemary, thyme)

In a small bowl, soak dried mushrooms in 1 cup hot water for 15 to 20 minutes. Drain, reserving the soaking liquid. Strain the liquid through a coffee filter; set aside. Rinse and chop the mushrooms.

Spray nonstick skillet with cooking spray. Add olive oil; heat. Add garlic and onion; sauté until translucent, about 3 minutes. Add peppers, herbs and seasoning; sauté another 30 seconds. Add fresh and soaked mushrooms; sauté until mushrooms soften, 3 to 4 minutes.

Pour the reserved soaking liquid into the skillet along with canned tomatoes and about half of the can's juice. Sauté, breaking up the tomatoes with a wooden spoon. Reduce heat to low and simmer about 5 minutes, until juices have been slightly reduced. Stir in parsley and cooked pasta, quickly tossing to coat pasta with sauce.

Sprinkle with Parmesan cheese and chopped herbs.

Serves 4.

Per Serving: 354 Calories

Protein 17 gr.	Carb. 54 gr.
Fat 8 gr.	Cal. from fat 21%
Chol. 67 mg.	Sodium 541 mg.

Squash Creole

1 tsp. olive oil
2 cloves garlic, minced
1 lb. yellow crookneck squash, cut into chunks
1 lb. zucchini squash, cut into chunks
1 red bell pepper, sliced thin lengthwise
1 tsp. Mrs. Dash seasoning
½ tsp. creole seasoning
1 Tbsp. chopped fresh herbs (cilantro, basil, rosemary, thyme)
¼ cup chicken stock (fat-free/low salt)

Spray a nonstick skillet with cooking spray; add the olive oil and heat. Add garlic and lightly sauté about 30 seconds. Add the squash, pepper, seasoning and herbs. Cook until squash is tender, stirring often, adding chicken stock to prevent sticking.

Serves 4.

Per Serving: 50 Calories

Protein 3 gr.	Carb. 8 gr.
Fat 1.5 gr.	Cal. from fat 24%
Chol. 0 mg.	Sodium 140 mg.

Risotto With Spring Vegetables

cheeses (protein)
rice (complex carb.)
vegetables, fruit (simple carb.)

Risotto With Spring Vegetables

5 ½ to 6 ½ cups chicken stock
    (fat-free/low salt)
16 baby carrots, shaved and cut in half
8 medium stalks asparagus, trimmed
    and cut into 2-inch pieces
1 cup sugar snap peas (thawed if frozen)
1 red bell pepper, cut into strips
2 tsp. olive oil
2 cloves garlic, minced
1 red onion, diced
1 cup arborio rice, uncooked
½ cup white wine*
½ tsp. creole seasoning
1 ½ Tbsp. chopped fresh basil
½ cup grated Parmesan cheese
2 Tbsp. chopped fresh herbs (cilantro,
    basil, rosemary, thyme)

* or substitute dealcoholized wine or more
  chicken stock

In medium-sized stockpot, bring chicken stock to boil over medium heat. Add carrots and cook 3 to 5 minutes until almost tender. Add asparagus, snap peas and pepper. Cook 1 minute longer. Remove vegetables with slotted spoon and place in bowl to cool. Reduce heat and keep stock simmering.

Spray a nonstick skillet with cooking spray. Add olive oil; heat. Add garlic and onions, and sauté until translucent, about 3 minutes. Add rice and stir to coat grains. Add wine and cook until most of liquid has been absorbed, about 2 to 3 minutes. Add ½ cup simmering chicken stock and cook another 2 to 3 minutes.

Continue adding stock, ½ cup at a time, until rice begins to soften, about 15 minutes.

Stir in the seasoning and basil, adding more stock to keep mixture creamy. Stir in reserved vegetables and cheese. Sprinkle with herbs.
Serves 4.

Per Serving: 316 Calories

Protein 13 gr.	Carb. 52 gr.
Fat 7 gr.	Cal. from fat 19%
Chol. 10 mg.	Sodium 393 mg.

Mixed Green Salad With Oranges

1 small red onion, sliced thin
2 navel oranges, peeled and sliced
4 cups washed, dried and torn mixed
    greens (red leaf, romaine,
    frizee, radicchio, arugula or bibb)
½ cup Balsamic Marinade (pg. 56)
1 cup whole-grain croutons (purchased)
¼ cup crumbled feta cheese

In a salad bowl, toss together all ingredients with dressing. Divide into fourths and serve on salad plates, allowing orange slices to remain on the top.
Serves 4.

Per Serving: 93 Calories

Protein 3.5 gr.	Carb. 14 gr.
Fat 2 gr.	Cal. from fat 20%
Chol. 6 mg.	Sodium 229 mg.

Try Risotto!

Risotto is a creamy, classic Northern Italian dish made with short-grain, highly starched rice, such as arborio.

Start risotto by sautéing rice in a small amount of olive oil for a few minutes until it is opaque.

Add hot liquid to rice ½ cup at a time, stirring constantly until the rice absorbs the liquid before adding more liquid.

Keep the broth over low heat, ready to be added. Stir in extra ingredients a few minutes before serving.

Risotto is wonderful made with wild mushrooms or saffron.

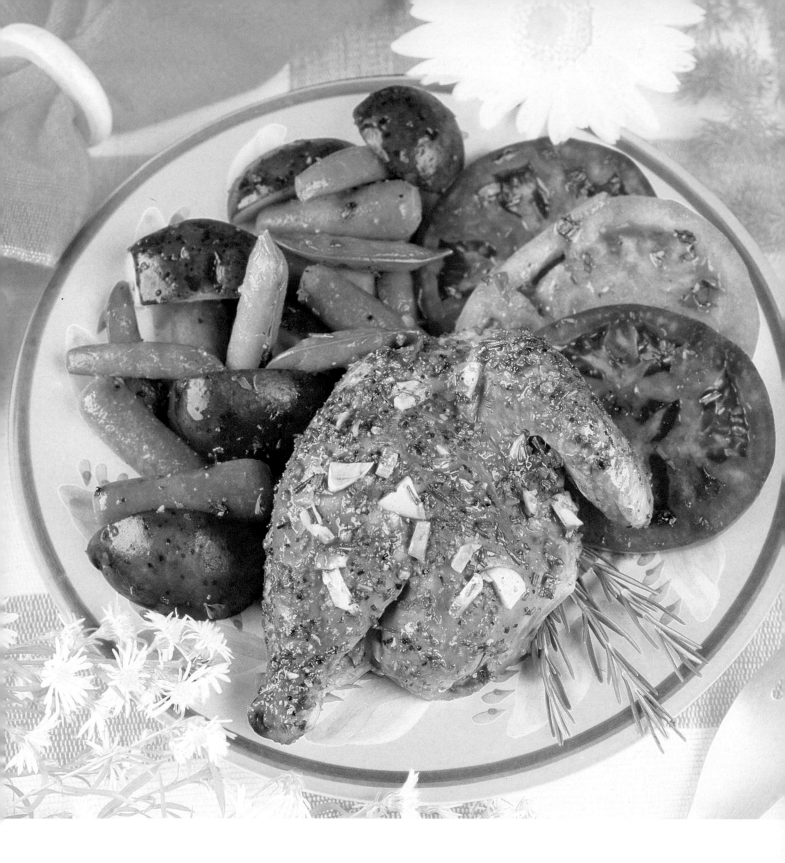

Home-style cooking is updated in this hearty menu with fresh and rustic flavor. The Cornish hens have been flavorfully marinated with herbs, then roasted to a golden brown. Served with marinated tomatoes on a bed of new potatoes, carrots and sugar snap peas, this is a simple and elegant meal that brings comfort and joy in any season.

Fresh Country Meal

game hens (protein)
potatoes (complex carb.)
carrots, snap peas, tomatoes (simple carb.)

Cornish Game Hens

2 Cornish hens, halved lengthwise
$^2/_3$ cup Lea and Perrins Worcestershire
    for Chicken
2 cloves garlic, minced
2 Tbsp. chopped fresh rosemary
1 tsp. Mrs. Dash seasoning
$^1/_2$ tsp. creole seasoning

Preheat oven to 375 degrees.
Remove skin from Cornish hens where possible. Place in small roasting pan and top with remaining ingredients. Let marinate for at least 1 hour.
Place hens in oven for 45 minutes or until juices run clear when pierced with fork. Brush occasionally with Worcestershire sauce in pan. See picture for beautiful plate presentation.
Serves 4.

Per Serving: 150 Calories

Protein 25 gr.	Carb. 0 gr.
Fat 4 gr.	Cal. from fat 28%
Chol. 74 mg.	Sodium 202 mg.

Marinated Tomatoes

4 tomatoes
$^1/_2$ cup Balsamic Marinade (pg. 56)
2 Tbsp. chopped fresh basil
1 tsp. cracked black pepper
$^1/_2$ tsp. creole seasoning

Slice each tomato into 5 to 7 slices and marinate in Balsamic Marinade for up to 1 hour. Sprinkle with basil, pepper and seasoning.
Serves 4.

Per Serving: 34 Calories

Protein 1 gr.	Carb. 5 gr.
Fat 1 gr.	Cal. from fat 26%
Chol. 0 mg.	Sodium 168 mg.

Sautéed Carrots and New Potatoes

1 lb. (8 to 10) small red-skinned
    potatoes, quartered
1 tsp. olive oil
2 cloves garlic, minced
1 cup baby carrots, shaved
$^1/_2$ tsp. Mrs. Dash seasoning
$^1/_2$ tsp. creole seasoning
1 Tbsp. chopped fresh herbs (cilantro,
    basil, rosemary, thyme)
$^1/_4$ cup chicken stock (fat-free/low salt)
$^1/_2$ lb. frozen sugar snap peas, thawed

Place red-skinned potatoes in microwaveable dish with $^1/_4$ cup water. Microwave on high power for 4 minutes; drain.
Spray a nonstick skillet with cooking spray, then add olive oil. Heat. Add garlic to pan; lightly sauté. Add potatoes, carrots, seasonings and herbs. Sauté for 5 minutes, adding chicken stock as needed; add sugar snap peas and sauté until crisp tender.
Serves 4.

Per Serving: 117 Calories

Protein 4 gr.	Carb. 23 gr.
Fat 1.5 gr.	Cal. from fat 11%
Chol. 0 mg.	Sodium 167 mg.

Zesty Fresh Herbs

Fresh herbs give pizzazz to a dish that dried herbs just can't match. They are easy to grow and easy to buy. Look for those with a clean, fresh fragrance and bright color. You can keep them for up to 5 days in the refrigerator by wrapping them loosely in a damp paper towel and sealing them airtight in a plastic bag.

Just before using herbs, wash them, then blot with a paper towel. Kitchen shears are great for snipping fresh herbs into small pieces.

Grilled Chicken Over Mixed Greens

chicken, beans (protein)
corn, beans (complex carb.)
greens (simple carb.)

Gourmet Secret: Marinating

Marinating low-fat meats and vegetables before grilling will help to keep them moist and full of flavor. When marinated meats hit the high heat of the grill, the outside is seared, sealing the flavor and moisture inside.

Vinegars, wines, fruit juices and yogurts are great main ingredients for low-fat marinades. Combine with garlic or shallots and your favorite herbs and spices for extra pizzazz.

Grilled Chicken Over Mixed Greens

½ cup Balsamic Marinade (pg. 56)
4 boneless, skinless chicken breast halves (1 lb.)
12 cups mixture of torn romaine, bibb and red leaf lettuces
1 cup Citrus Vinaigrette (pg. 52)
2 Tbsp. chopped fresh herbs (cilantro, basil, rosemary, thyme)
3 tomatoes, cut into quarters

Marinate the chicken breasts in Balsamic Marinade for at least 1 hour. Grill, or sear in hot skillet, basting with marinade to keep moist.

Toss lettuce mixture with Citrus Vinaigrette. Place grilled chicken on top and sprinkle all with chopped herbs.

Garnish with tomato quarters.

Serves 4.

Per Serving: 259 Calories

Protein 31 gr.	Carb. 18 gr.
Fat 7 gr.	Cal. from fat 24%
Chol. 72 mg.	Sodium 248 mg.

Black Bean and Corn Salsa

1 can (16 oz.) or 2 cups black beans, drained and rinsed
8 oz. frozen corn kernels, thawed
2 plum tomatoes, diced
½ red onion, minced
1 serrano or jalapeño pepper, seeded and minced
1 Tbsp. finely chopped cilantro
1 Tbsp. olive oil
4 cloves garlic, minced
juice of 1 lime
1 Tbsp. balsamic vinegar
1 tsp. cumin
2 tsp. hot pepper sauce
1 tsp. creole seasoning

In a large bowl, combine all ingredients and mix well. Allow to marinate at least one hour. Makes 10 servings, ⅓ cup each.

Per Serving: 79 Calories

Protein 4 gr.	Carb. 13 gr.
Fat 1.5 gr.	Cal. from fat 17%
Chol. 0 mg.	Sodium 118 mg.

Breast of Chicken Nicoise

chicken (protein)
couscous (complex carb.)
vegetables (simple carb.)

Breast of Chicken Nicoise

4 boneless, skinless chicken breast
   halves (1 lb.)
1 tsp. Mrs. Dash garlic herb seasoning,
   divided
1 tsp. creole seasoning, divided
½ cup fennel, cut into strips
½ cup leeks, cut into strips
1 tsp. olive oil
2 cloves garlic, minced
½ cup cucumber, cut in strips
1½ cups chicken stock (fat-free/low salt)
½ cup white wine*
1 large tomato, seeded and cut into
   strips
¼ cup chopped fresh basil leaves
8 Nicoise olives, quartered
2 Tbsp. chopped fresh parsley

*   or substitute dealcoholized wine or more
    chicken stock

Clean chicken breasts of all fat and tendons.
Season with ½ tsp. Mrs. Dash and ⅛ tsp. creole seasoning. Grill, or sear in hot skillet, on each
side until done.

Meanwhile, steam fennel and leeks. Spray
sauté pan with cooking spray; add olive oil and
heat. Add garlic and quickly sauté. Add steamed
vegetables and cucumber, and quickly sauté.
Add chicken stock and wine, then add tomato,
remaining seasonings, basil and olives. Simmer
until reduced by half.

Place grilled chicken breasts on plate.
Sprinkle with chopped parsley. Cover with veg-
etables and sauce.
   Serves 4.

Per Serving: 209 Calories

Protein 28 gr.	Carb. 11 gr.
Fat 6 gr.	Cal. from fat 25%
Chol. 72 mg.	Sodium 384 mg.

Herbed Couscous

1¼ cups chicken stock (fat-free/low salt)
1 tsp. olive oil
½ tsp. Tabasco
¼ tsp. salt
1 tsp. Mrs. Dash seasoning
1 cup quick-cooking couscous
1 Tbsp. chopped fresh parsley
⅛ tsp. cracked black pepper

In small saucepan, combine chicken stock,
olive oil, Tabasco, salt and seasoning, and bring
to a boil. Stir in couscous and remove from heat.
Cover with a tight-fitting lid and let stand for
5 minutes. Uncover and fluff with fork to separate. Stir in parsley and pepper.
   Serves 4.

Per Serving: 183 Calories

Protein 5 gr.	Carb. 35 gr.
Fat 1 gr.	Cal. from fat 7%
Chol. 0 mg.	Sodium 141 mg.

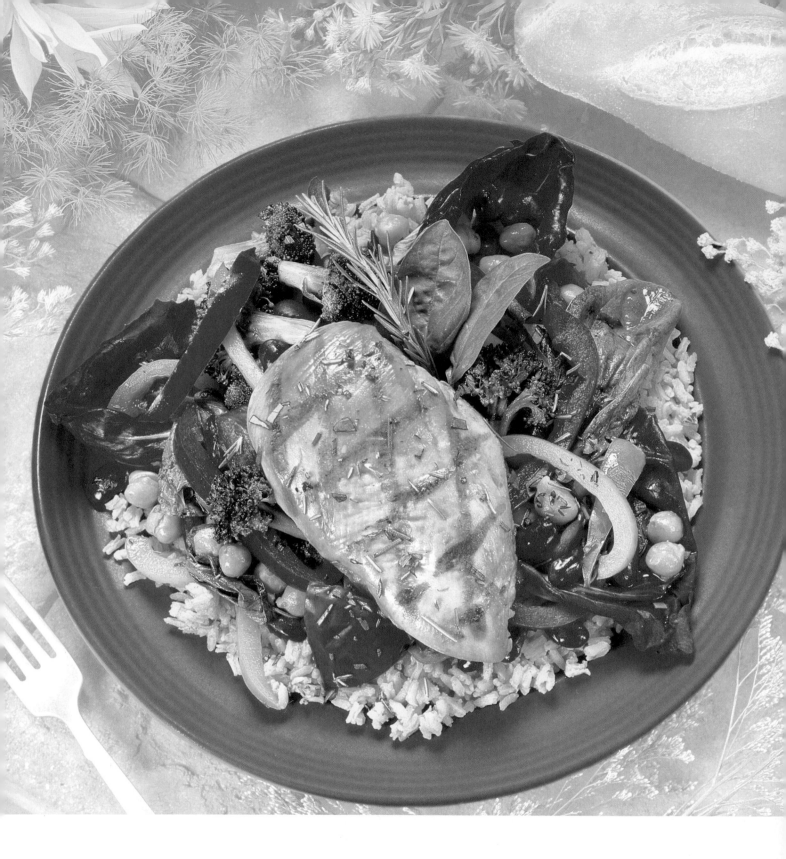

Inspired by a creation of Marco Barbitta, chef and owner of the Trading Post Cafe in Taos, New Mexico, this dish is a delightful blend of flavors, colors and textures. The vegetables are quickly sautéed in a tasty herbal broth and served atop vibrant saffron rice. The marinated grilled breast of chicken is the crowning touch!

Chicken Marco

chicken (protein)
rice (complex carb.)
vegetables (simple carb.)

Chicken Marco

²⁄₃ cup Balsamic Marinade (pg. 56)
4 boneless, skinless chicken breast
   halves (1 lb.)
2 cloves garlic, minced
2 tsp. shallots, minced
1 cup broccoli florets, blanched
1 each red, green and yellow pepper,
   cut into strips
1½ cups red beans, cooked and
   drained
1½ cups chickpeas, cooked and
   drained
2 plum tomatoes, cut into quarters
1 cup chicken stock (fat-free/low salt)
1 cup white wine*
1 tsp. creole seasoning
1 tsp. Mrs. Dash seasoning
2 Tbsp. chopped fresh herbs (cilantro,
   basil, rosemary, thyme)
2 cups fresh spinach leaves, washed
   and stemmed
12 radicchio leaves

* or substitute dealcoholized wine or more
  chicken stock

Marinate chicken breasts in Balsamic Marinade for at least 1 hour. Grill chicken breasts until done.

Spray a nonstick skillet with cooking spray. Heat. Add garlic and shallots to pan; lightly sauté. Add blanched broccoli, peppers, beans, chickpeas, tomatoes, chicken stock, wine, seasonings and herbs. Lightly sauté, allowing liquid to reduce. Add spinach and radicchio at end of cooking to allow to wilt with heat.

To serve, spoon ½ cup saffron rice onto each plate. Top with a fourth of sautéed vegetable mixture. Add a grilled chicken breast, and spoon skillet broth over chicken and rice.

Serves 4.

Per Serving: 371 Calories

Protein 41 gr.	Carb. 42 gr.
Fat 6 gr.	Cal. from fat 14%
Chol. 72 mg.	Sodium 559 mg.

Saffron Rice

1 tsp. olive oil
2 cloves garlic, minced
1¾ cups chicken stock (fat-free/low salt)
4 to 5 saffron threads (or ¼ tsp. powder)
⅛ tsp. cumin
½ tsp. creole seasoning
1 Tbsp. chopped fresh parsley
   (or 1 tsp. dried)
2 cups instant brown rice

Spray a medium saucepan with cooking spray; add olive oil and heat. Add minced garlic and lightly sauté about 1 to 2 minutes, then add chicken stock, saffron, cumin, seasoning and parsley. Let come to a boil, then stir in brown rice. Boil for 1 minute, turn down heat to low and cover. Simmer for 5 minutes; uncover saucepan and fluff rice with fork. Cover again, and let sit for another 5 minutes.

Serves 4.

Per Serving: 126 Calories

Protein 2.5 gr.	Carb. 24 gr.
Fat 2 gr.	Cal. from fat 15%
Chol. 0 mg.	Sodium 136 mg.

The Saffron Secret

Saffron is the world's most expensive spice. You can buy it in threads or powder, or in a less expensive "imitation" form such as turmeric. The powder loses its flavor easily and should be bought in very small quantities. That's all anyone can afford, anyway!

When using the threads, crush just before using. Heat will release saffron's flavor essence, so mixing it with 1 Tbsp. of very hot water and letting it stand for 10 minutes will increase its impact.

Chicken Curry Over Rice

chicken (protein)
rice (complex carb.)
cucumber (simple carb.)

Coconut Milk

Canned, unsweetened coconut milk—not to be confused with the sweetened coconut "cream" used in sweet drinks—can be found in your supermarket's Asian food section or in a specialty market. It is made from simmering coconut "meat" in water. It adds a subtle flavor and silky texture to many soups and sauces.

Chicken Curry Over Rice

¼ cup unsweetened coconut milk
2 tsp. cornstarch
1 lb. boneless, skinless chicken breasts
½ tsp. creole seasoning
1 tsp. canola oil
1 small onion, chopped
1 red bell pepper, cored, seeded and julienned
2 cloves garlic, minced
1 jalapeño pepper, seeded and finely chopped
4 tsp. curry powder
1 tsp. cumin
1 tsp. ground coriander
1 cup evaporated skim milk
juice of 1 lime
¼ cup chopped fresh cilantro
2 cups brown rice, cooked

In a small bowl, whisk together coconut milk and cornstarch until smooth; set aside.

Spray a large, heavy saucepan with cooking spray and heat over medium heat. Cut chicken into 2-inch chunks and season with creole seasoning. Add to saucepan, quickly sautéing until browned. Remove chicken from pan and set aside.

To same saucepan, add canola oil, onion and red bell pepper, reserving a few pieces of pepper for garnish; sauté until softened, about 5 minutes. Add garlic, jalapeño pepper, curry powder, cumin and coriander; sauté about 2 minutes more.

Reduce heat to low and stir in coconut milk mixture and evaporated skim milk. Bring to a simmer, stirring. Cook for another 5 minutes, then add chicken. Heat through, stirring in lime juice and cilantro. Serve over brown rice. Garnish with reserved red pepper.

Serves 4.

Per Serving: 359 Calories

Protein 35 gr.	Carb. 34 gr.
Fat 8 gr.	Cal. from fat 23%
Chol. 74 mg.	Sodium 278 mg.

Chilled Cucumber Salad

2 cucumbers (European, if available)
2 Tbsp. rice wine vinegar
½ tsp. sugar
½ tsp. creole seasoning
1 tsp. Mrs. Dash seasoning
1 Tbsp. fresh chopped dill
  (or 1 tsp. dried)

Peel cucumbers and cut in half lengthwise. With a teaspoon, scrape out and discard seeds. Cut the cucumbers crosswise into ¼-inch slices.

Place in a medium-size bowl along with the vinegar, sugar, seasonings and dill. Toss to combine and refrigerate until serving time.

Serves 4.

Per Serving: 21 Calories

Protein 1 gr.	Carb. 5 gr.
Fat 0 gr.	Cal. from fat 0%
Chol. 0 mg.	Sodium 137 mg.

Chicken Paella

chicken (protein)
rice, peas (complex carb.)
spinach salad (simple carb.)

Chicken Paella

1 lb. boneless, skinless chicken breast,
  trimmed of fat and cut into chunks
¼ cup Lea and Perrins Worcestershire
  for Chicken
2 tsp. olive oil
2 cloves garlic, minced
1 small onion, diced
1 cup arborio (or medium-grain) rice
2 cups chicken stock (fat-free/low salt)
¼ tsp. crushed saffron threads
  (or ⅛ tsp. powdered)
½ tsp. creole seasoning
1 tsp. Mrs. Dash seasoning
1 cup frozen peas, thawed
⅓ cup jarred, roasted red peppers,
  drained and cut into strips

Marinate chicken breasts in Worcestershire sauce for up to 1 hour.

Spray a large nonstick skillet with cooking spray. Add olive oil and heat over medium-high heat. Add garlic and onion, and sauté 30 seconds; then add marinated chicken chunks. Sauté until slightly browned on the outside and opaque inside, 3 to 4 minutes. Remove chicken from skillet and set aside.

To skillet, add rice; stir to coat well. Stir in chicken stock, saffron and seasonings. Cover and cook over low heat for 20 minutes. Gently stir in cooked chicken, green peas and roasted red peppers. Cover again and cook, stirring occasionally, until rice is tender, about 5 minutes more. Serve immediately.

Serves 4.

Per Serving: 414 Calories

Protein 32 gr.	Carb. 55 gr.
Fat 6 gr.	Cal. from fat 13%
Chol. 72 mg.	Sodium 616 mg.

Spinach Salad With Horseradish Dressing

12 oz. fresh spinach, washed and
  stemmed
½ cup grated carrots
½ cup grated zucchini
½ red onion, sliced thin
1 cup Horseradish Dressing (pg. 53)

Dry spinach in a salad spinner or on a towel. Toss all remaining ingredients together with dressing and spinach.

Serves 4.

Per Serving: 84 Calories

Protein 5 gr.	Carb. 16 gr.
Fat 0 gr.	Cal. from fat 0 %
Chol. 0 mg.	Sodium 176 mg.

Superior Spinach

Choose spinach leaves that are small, firm and dark green; if purchasing spinach by the bag, look for one marked "baby" or "salad" spinach.

To prepare, first discard any leaves that are wilted or discolored. Soak the spinach twice, holding the leaves by the stem and gently swishing the leaves underwater. Stem the spinach by folding each leaf lengthwise, then holding it in one hand, rib side out, and with the other hand pulling the stem off the leaf. Dry the spinach in a salad spinner or by wrapping the leaves in paper towels.

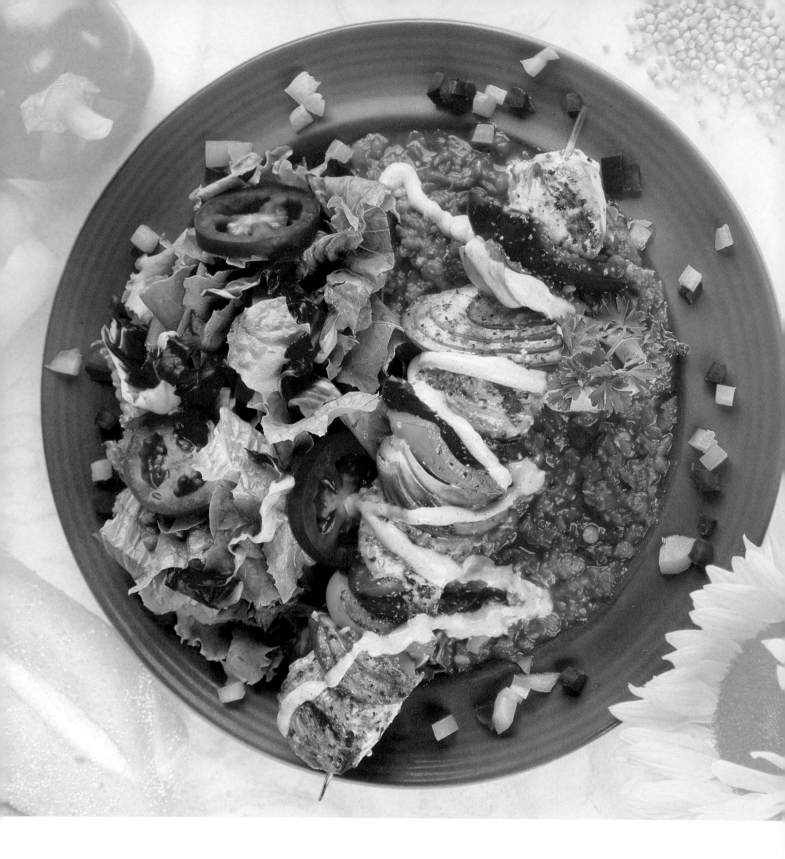

It sounds nouvelle, but chicken and lentils are actually a centuries-old pairing. Simmered with vegetables, the lentils make a rich bed for the chicken breast and red peppers, which are gently placed on top. If they're available, the red or French lentils give the dish a more delicate flavor.

Taste of India Dinner

chicken, lentils (protein)
lentils (complex carb.)
vegetables (simple carb.)

Chicken and Sweet Pepper Brochettes

4 wooden skewers
1 lb. boneless, skinless chicken breast, cut into large chunks
2 red bell peppers, cut into 12 chunks
2 yellow bell peppers, cut into 12 chunks
1 onion, cut into 12 pieces
½ cup Balsamic Marinade (pg. 56)
½ tsp. Mrs. Dash seasoning
1 tsp. creole seasoning
½ cup Yogurt Sauce (right column)
2 tsp. chopped fresh cilantro

• Serve with a green salad.

Skewer chunks of chicken and vegetables onto wooden skewers that have been soaked in water. Marinate in Balsamic Marinade for at least 1 hour or up to overnight. Sprinkle with seasonings and grill over hot coals.

Make a bed of Seasoned Lentil Sauté in the center of each of four plates. Place grilled skewers on top. Add a tablespoon of Yogurt Sauce and sprinkle with chopped cilantro.
Serves 4.

Per Serving: 203 Calories

Protein 31 gr.
Fat 3.5 gr.
Chol. 73 mg.

Carb. 11 gr.
Cal. from fat 16%
Sodium 377 mg.

Seasoned Lentil Sauté

1 Tbsp. shallots, chopped
2 cloves garlic, minced
2 cups red or brown lentils, cooked in chicken stock (fat-free/low salt)
½ cup red bell pepper, finely minced
½ cup yellow bell pepper, finely minced
1 tsp. Mrs. Dash seasoning
½ tsp. creole seasoning
1 cup white wine*
2 cups chicken stock (fat-free/low salt)

* or substitute dealcoholized wine or more chicken stock

Spray nonstick pan with cooking spray; heat. Add shallots and garlic; heat through. Add lentils, peppers, seasonings, wine and chicken stock. Gently cook until heated through and chicken stock is reduced slightly.
Serves 4.

Per Serving: 118 Calories

Protein 8 gr.
Fat 0 gr.
Chol. 0 mg.

Carb. 22 gr.
Cal. from fat 0%
Sodium 165 mg.

Savory Yogurt Sauce

This sauce is a flavorful topping to grilled meats. Put into a squirt bottle and get creative.

1 cup nonfat plain yogurt
2 Tbsp. skim milk
2 Tbsp. white wine*
juice of 1 lime
2 Tbsp. Dijon mustard
1 Tbsp. honey
1½ tsp. curry
1 tsp. turmeric
½ Tbsp. Mrs. Dash seasoning
1 Tbsp. chopped cilantro
1 tsp. chopped fresh mint

Combine all ingredients in a blender. Chill.

* or substitute dealcoholized wine or chicken stock

Chicken Laurent

chicken (protein)
rice (complex carb.)
asparagus, red onion (simple carb.)

What Are Shallots?

Shallots taste like a combination of onion and garlic, but are milder than both. They are formed more like garlic than onion, with a head comprised of multiple cloves, each covered with a thin, papery skin. Choose shallots that are plump and firm with dry skins. Avoid those that are wrinkled or sprouting. Store in a cool, dry, well-ventilated place for up to one month.

When a recipe calls for one shallot, it usually means one clove, not the whole head.

Chicken Laurent

4 boneless, skinless chicken
   breast halves (1 lb.)
¼ cup Lea and Perrins Worcestershire
   for Chicken
1 lb. asparagus, trimmed
2 tsp. olive oil
2 cloves garlic, minced
2 tsp. shallots, minced
1 tsp. Mrs. Dash seasoning
½ tsp. creole seasoning
1 red onion, sliced thin
⅓ cup white wine*
⅔ cup chicken stock (fat-free/low salt)
2 tsp. cornstarch

* or substitute dealcoholized wine or more
   chicken stock

Preheat oven to 375 degrees.
Marinate chicken breasts in Worcestershire sauce for at least 15 minutes.
Place asparagus spears with ¼ cup water in a glass baking dish; cover with vented plastic wrap. Microwave on high to blanch for 3 to 4 minutes.
Spray nonstick ovenproof skillet with cooking spray. Add olive oil and heat. Add garlic and shallots to pan; lightly sauté. Add marinated chicken breasts and brown on both sides, sprinkling with seasonings. Lay asparagus and red onion slices on top of chicken.
Stir together wine and chicken stock in a small stock pot; add cornstarch mixed with 1 Tbsp. cold water. Stir over moderate heat until thickened. Pour over chicken and vegetables.
Bake in oven for 30 minutes.
Serves 4.

Per Serving: 214 Calories

Protein 30 gr.	Carb. 11 gr.
Fat 6 gr.	Cal. from fat 24%
Chol. 72 mg.	Sodium 338 mg.

Quick Brown Rice Pilaf

1 tsp. olive oil
½ red onion, diced
2 cloves garlic, minced
1¾ cups chicken stock (fat-free/low salt)
½ tsp. creole seasoning
1 Tbsp. chopped fresh herbs (cilantro,
   basil, rosemary, thyme)
2 cups instant brown rice

Spray a medium saucepan with cooking spray; add olive oil and heat. Add diced onion and garlic, and lightly sauté about 1 to 2 minutes; then add chicken stock, seasoning and herbs.
Let mixture come to a boil, then stir in brown rice. Let boil for 1 minute, turn down heat to low and cover. Let simmer for 5 minutes, uncover skillet and fluff rice with fork. Cover again. Let sit for another 5 minutes.
Serves 6.

Per Serving: 126 Calories

Protein 2.5 gr.	Carb. 24 gr.
Fat 2 gr.	Cal. from fat 15%
Chol. 0 mg.	Sodium 136 mg.

Turkey Carbonara

turkey, cheeses (protein)
pasta (complex carb.)
vegetables, fruit (simple carb.)

Turkey Carbonara

8 oz. dried linguine, preferably whole wheat
2 strips turkey bacon, chopped
1 shallot, minced
2 cloves garlic, minced
8 oz. smoked turkey, cut into chunks
½ cup frozen green peas, thawed
2 Tbsp. chopped fresh herbs (cilantro, basil, rosemary, thyme)
2 cups Carbonara Sauce
1 tsp. Mrs. Dash seasoning
½ tsp. creole seasoning
2 Tbsp. chopped fresh basil
1 plum tomato, diced

- Serve with a green salad and ½ cup chopped mixed fruit.

In a large stockpot, cook pasta in boiling salted water until done, preferably al dente (slightly firm). Set aside.

Spray large sauté pan with cooking spray; heat. Add turkey bacon pieces, then shallots and garlic. Begin to cook over low heat. Add smoked turkey.

Add pasta, peas and fresh herbs, and sauté quickly. Then add Carbonara Sauce. Bring to a simmer and add seasonings. Serve immediately, sprinkled with basil and tomato.

Serves 4.

Per Serving: 383 Calories

Protein 33 gr.	Carb. 40 gr.
Fat 9 gr.	Cal. from fat 22%
Chol. 86 mg.	Sodium 537 mg.

Carbonara Sauce

1 Tbsp. olive oil
2 Tbsp. all-purpose or whole-wheat flour
2 cups skim milk
¼ cup white wine*
¼ cup skim-milk ricotta cheese
1 tsp. Mrs. Dash garlic herb seasoning
½ tsp. creole seasoning
¼ cup grated Parmesan cheese

* or substitute dealcoholized wine or chicken stock (fat-free/low salt)

Spray a nonstick skillet with cooking spray. Add olive oil and heat. Add flour, stirring with oil until blended.

Add skim milk; bring to a boil and simmer slowly until thickened, stirring often. Add white wine, ricotta and seasonings. Stir over low heat until smooth. Stir in Parmesan cheese.

Makes 6 servings, ¾ cup each.

Per Serving: 79 Calories

Protein 8 gr.	Carb. 5.5 gr.
Fat 2.5 gr.	Cal. from fat 29%
Chol. 4 mg.	Sodium 215 mg.

Cooking Cheeses

Cheese can turn stringy, rubbery or grainy when exposed to high heat. Avoid this by first shredding or cutting cheese into small pieces and stirring into the sauce toward the end of cooking. Cook over low heat until cheese melts. Low-fat cheeses will melt more slowly than traditional ones; be gentle!

dinners

Turkey With a Thai Twist

turkey (protein)
waffles (complex carb.)
broccoli, tomatoes (simple carb.)

Corn Waffles With Turkey Breast Cutlets

4 turkey breast cutlets (1 lb.)
½ cup Balsamic Marinade (pg. 56)
12 oz. purchased whole-wheat
    pancake or waffle mix (or
    Homemade Pancake Mix, pg. 78)
2 cups frozen corn kernels, thawed
2 Tbsp. chopped chives
1 cup Thai Dressing
2 cups broccoli florets, cooked
1 red pepper, minced
12 tomato slices (about 2 large
    tomatoes)

Clean turkey cutlets of skin and fat. Marinate in Balsamic Marinade overnight. Grill turkey. Set aside.

Spray waffle iron with cooking spray. Prepare waffle mix according to package directions; add corn and chives. Cook in waffle iron 3 to 5 minutes, until golden brown and cooked through.

Place one waffle and one turkey cutlet on each of four plates. Drizzle Thai Dressing over the turkey. Place broccoli on plate. Sprinkle all with minced pepper. Serve with sliced tomatoes.

    Serves 4.

Thai Dressing

¾ cup lime juice
¾ cup chicken stock (fat-free/low salt)
½ cup honey
¼ cup fish sauce*
1 Tbsp. oyster sauce*
1 tsp. chili sauce
2 Tbsp. grated fresh ginger
3 Tbsp. chopped fresh cilantro

* *These are found in the Oriental
   section of your grocery store.*

Combine all ingredients in a blender.
Use additional dressing to create an exotic Oriental salad for another night. Dressing will keep refrigerated up to 2 weeks.
Makes 10 servings, ¼ cup each.

Per Serving: 65 Calories

Protein 0 gr.	Carb. 16 gr.
Fat 0 gr.	Cal. from fat 0%
Chol. 0 mg.	Sodium 216 mg.

Chicken Au Poivre

chicken (protein)
orzo (complex carb.)
vegetables (simple carb.)

Chicken Au Poivre

4 boneless, skinless chicken breast
    halves (1 lb.)
1 tsp. cracked black pepper
½ tsp. Mrs. Dash seasoning
1 tsp. olive oil
2 cloves garlic, minced
1 small red onion, finely chopped
¼ cup fennel, sliced into
    ½-inch slices
¼ cup sun-dried tomatoes, slivered
2 tsp. capers, rinsed
2 cups cooked orzo
2 shiitake mushrooms, sliced
1 cup white wine*
2 cups chicken stock (fat-free/low salt)
2 Tbsp. lemon juice
4 basil leaves
1 tsp. creole seasoning

*   or substitute dealcoholized wine or more
    chicken stock

Rub chicken with pepper and Mrs. Dash. Grill over hot coals, or sear in hot skillet until done. Set aside.

Spray nonstick skillet with cooking spray. Add olive oil and heat on medium high. Sauté garlic, onion and fennel until all begin to soften, about 3 to 4 minutes. Add sun-dried tomatoes, capers and orzo; stir. Add mushrooms, white wine, chicken stock, lemon juice, basil and creole seasoning. Cook gently for another 3 to 4 minutes or until liquids begin to reduce. Pour entire mixture, including juice, onto plate.

Top with the grilled chicken and 1 Tbsp. of Basil Sauce per serving.

Serves 4.

Per Serving: 340 Calories

Protein 32 gr.	Carb. 36 gr.
Fat 7.5 gr.	Cal. from fat 20%
Chol. 72 mg.	Sodium 820 mg.

Basil Sauce

½ cup white wine*
2 Tbsp. chopped fresh basil
2 Tbsp. lemon juice
½ tsp. cracked black pepper

*   or substitute dealcoholized wine or
    chicken stock (fat-free/low salt)

Mix together all ingredients.
Makes 10 servings, 1 Tbsp. each.

Per Serving: 9 Calories

Protein 0 gr.	Carb. 2 gr.
Fat 0 gr.	Cal. from fat 0%
Chol. 0 mg.	Sodium 7 mg.

Flavorful Fresh Fennel

Fresh fennel has a broad, bulb-shaped base with celery-like stems and bright green leaves. The aromatic and flavorful bulbs and stems can be used raw in salads or cooked in a variety of ways: braised, sautéed, boiled or marinated and grilled. The greenery can be used as a garnish or snipped and used as a last-minute flavor enhancer.

Favorite Summer BBQ

chicken (protein)
corn (complex carb.)
cabbage, apple, mango (simple carb.)

Cooking Corn in the Husk

Corn is best and sweetest when cooked in the husks. Gently pull back the husks, remove the silk, then replace the husks, tying them together at the top with a string or a strip of the husk itself. Cook as you would husked corn, even when boiling. Don't overcook the corn, or it will get tougher, as it will if cooked in salted water.

When grilling corn, soak the corn in cold water for 15 minutes so that the husks don't burn while grilling. As an alternative, microwave for 4 to 5 minutes before grilling to greatly reduce cooking time.

BBQ Breast of Chicken

4 boneless, skinless chicken breast
   halves (1 lb.)
½ cup Jamaican Marinade (pg. 57)
1 cup Citrus BBQ sauce (pg. 56)
1⅓ cups Apple Chutney

Marinate chicken breasts in Jamaican Marinade for at least 1 hour. Grill, basting with Citrus BBQ sauce. Serve over Apple Chutney.
   Serves 4.

Per Serving: 252 Calories

Protein 28 gr.	Carb. 26 gr.
Fat 4 gr.	Cal. from fat 14%
Chol. 72 mg.	Sodium 410 mg.

Tricolor Coleslaw

2 cups red cabbage, shredded
2 cups green cabbage, shredded
1 cup carrots, grated
½ cup Citrus Vinaigrette (pg. 52)
2 Tbsp. chopped fresh herbs (cilantro,
   basil, rosemary, thyme)
½ tsp. creole seasoning
1 tsp. Mrs. Dash seasoning

In a large bowl, combine all ingredients, tossing well. Refrigerate until chilled.
   Serves 4.

Per Serving: 49 Calories

Protein 1 gr.	Carb. 8 gr.
Fat 1.5 gr.	Cal. from fat 29%
Chol. 1 mg.	Sodium 273 mg.

Grilled Corn on the Cob

4 ears of corn (with husks intact)

Carefully peel back husks but do not detach. Remove silk; replace the husks back over the corn (leave a small bit exposed) and secure the top by pulling two pieces of husk to the front and tying into a bow-tie knot.
   Microwave on high for 4 minutes.
   Place exposed side of the corn on the grill, periodically turning for even cooking, until the ears are tender when pierced, about 8 minutes.
   Serves 4.

Per Serving: 83 Calories

Protein 2 gr.	Carb. 19 gr.
Fat 0 gr.	Cal. from fat 0%
Chol. 0 mg.	Sodium 13 mg.

Apple Chutney

1 Granny Smith apple, thinly julienned
1 cup Mango Chutney (pg. 62)

Mix together and refrigerate to blend flavors. Makes 4 servings, ⅓ cup each.

Per Serving: 47 Calories

Protein 0 gr.	Carb. 12 gr.
Fat 0 gr.	Cal. from fat 0%
Chol. 0 mg.	Sodium 272 mg.

Veal Picatta

veal (protein)
orzo (complex carb.)
squash (simple carb.)

Veal Picatta

4 slices veal, about 1 inch thick (1 lb.)*
¼ cup Lea and Perrins Worcestershire
    for Chicken
⅓ cup all-purpose flour
1 tsp. Mrs. Dash seasoning, divided
1 tsp. creole seasoning, divided
2 tsp. olive oil
2 cloves garlic, minced
2 Tbsp. chopped fresh herbs (cilantro,
    basil, rosemary, thyme)
½ cup chicken stock (fat-free/low salt)
1 lemon, peeled and cut into segments
½ tsp. sugar
1 Tbsp. capers, rinsed

* *may substitute pork cutlets, trimmed of fat*

• **Serve with Squash Creole (pg. 108).**

Pound veal slices to tenderize. Marinate in Worcestershire sauce up to 1 hour.

Combine flour, ½ tsp. Mrs. Dash and ½ tsp. creole seasoning in a shallow dish. Lightly dredge marinated veal slices in the flour mixture, shaking off the excess.

Spray a nonstick skillet with cooking spray, then add olive oil; heat. Add the veal to the pan and cook until the outside is golden brown, about 2 to 3 minutes each side. Transfer to a platter and keep warm. Add garlic to the same skillet; lightly sauté. Add remaining seasonings and herbs; then stir in more chicken stock and bring to a boil. Stir while cooking for 1 minute.

Add lemon segments, sugar and capers; cook for 30 seconds more.

Serves 4.

Per Serving: 212 Calories

Protein 24 gr.	Carb. 11 gr.
Fat 7 gr.	Cal. from fat 32%
Chol. 93 mg.	Sodium 401 mg.

Herbed Orzo

8 oz. package of orzo
1 tsp. olive oil
2 cloves garlic, minced
½ cup chicken stock (fat-free/low salt)
½ tsp. creole seasoning
1 tsp. Mrs. Dash seasoning
1 tsp. chopped fresh basil

In a large stockpot, cook orzo in salted water according to package directions until done.

Spray a nonstick skillet with cooking spray, then add olive oil. Heat. Add garlic and sauté for 30 seconds. Then add remaining ingredients and cooked orzo, lightly sautéing to coat. Serve immediately.

Serves 6.

Per Serving: 101 Calories

Protein 2 gr.	Carb. 21 gr.
Fat 1 gr.	Cal. from fat 9%
Chol. 0 mg.	Sodium 141 mg.

Grilled Sirloin and New Potato Salad

steak (protein)
potatoes, toast (complex carb.)
peppers, greens (simple carb.)

Shop Smart for Meat

When buying meat, all cuts should be lean and trimmed of visible fat. The leanest cuts of beef and veal are the round, loin, sirloin and extra-lean ground beef. The leanest pork is from the tenderloin, leg and shoulder. The leanest lamb is from the leg, loin and rib. Poultry should be skinless.

Grilled Sirloin and New Potato Salad

⅓ cup Balsamic Marinade (pg. 56)
¾ lb. lean sirloin*, trimmed of all fat
2 red bell peppers, cut in half lengthwise
1 large red onion, cut into thick slices
8 red-skinned potatoes, halved
½ tsp. creole seasoning
½ tsp. Mrs. Dash seasoning
12 cups washed, dried and torn mixed greens (red leaf, romaine, frizee, radicchio, arugula or bibb)
½ cup Honey-Orange Vinaigrette (pg. 51)
2 Tbsp. chopped fresh herbs (cilantro, basil, rosemary, thyme)

* *may use skinless, boneless chicken breasts*

Marinate meat, peppers and onion in Balsamic Marinade for up to 3 hours.

Microwave potatoes and ¼ cup water in a glass dish, covered with plastic wrap (vented) on high for 4 minutes.

Carefully place meat, cooked potatoes and other vegetables on grill and sprinkle with seasonings. Cook for 4 minutes. Turn over meat and vegetables, and cook until the meat is done and vegetables are slightly charred, about another 3 to 4 minutes. Slice the grilled peppers and sirloin into strips and toss with other grilled vegetables, lettuces and Honey-Orange Vinaigrette.

Serves 4.

Per Serving: 329 Calories

Protein 25 gr.	Carb. 41 gr.
Fat 8 gr.	Cal. from fat 22%
Chol. 57 mg.	Sodium 249 mg.

Garlic Toast

4 slices (½-inch thick) French, Italian or sourdough bread
garlic-flavored cooking spray
1 large garlic clove, cut in half
¼ cup Balsamic Marinade (pg. 56)

Prepare a grill. Spray the bread slices with garlic-flavored cooking spray and place on grill. Grill bread, turning once, until well toasted on both sides, about 2 to 3 minutes per side. Rub one side of each slice with the cut side of the garlic clove and brush with Balsamic Marinade.

Serves 4.

Per Serving: 93 Calories

Protein 3 gr.	Carb. 18 gr.
Fat 1 gr.	Cal. from fat 10%
Chol. 0 mg.	Sodium 214 mg.

Beef Stew

beef (protein)
bread (complex carb.)
vegetables (simple carb.)

Beef Stew

1 lb. top sirloin of beef, trimmed
   of all fat and cut into chunks
¼ cup Balsamic Marinade (pg. 56)
¼ lb. baby carrots, shaved
1 zucchini, cut into ½-inch slices
1 cup green beans, trimmed
1 tsp. Mrs. Dash seasoning, divided
1 tsp. creole seasoning, divided
1 red onion, chopped
1 cup red wine*
1½ cups beef stock (fat-free/low salt)
1 Tbsp. chopped fresh basil
1 tsp. dried crushed thyme
¼ tsp. crushed black pepper
2 whole plum tomatoes, quartered
1 Tbsp. chopped fresh chives

* or substitute dealcoholized wine or beef
  stock (fat-free/low salt)

Marinate beef overnight in Balsamic Marinade.

In a large saucepot, place carrots, zucchini and green beans with ½ cup water. Steam for 7 to 8 minutes or until crisp tender.

Season beef with ½ tsp. Mrs. Dash and ½ tsp. creole seasoning. Spray nonstick skillet with cooking spray. Sear beef with onions in the hot skillet. Add red wine and stir; then remove beef. To the same skillet, add steamed vegetables, beef stock, basil, thyme, pepper and remaining seasonings.

Simmer over medium-high heat until liquid is reduced about halfway. Add beef back to pan and sauté quickly to heat through. Add tomatoes. Sprinkle with fresh chives when serving.

Serves 4.

Per Serving: 261 Calories

Protein 29 gr.	Carb. 16 gr.
Fat 9 gr.	Cal. from fat 32%
Chol. 76 mg.	Sodium 354 mg.

Chopped Tomato Salad With Garlic Toast

2 medium ripe tomatoes, chopped
1 medium red bell pepper, chopped
1 medium yellow bell pepper, chopped
1 small red onion, chopped
2 tsp. capers
3 Tbsp. chopped fresh basil
1 Tbsp. balsamic vinegar
2 tsp. freshly squeezed lemon juice
2 cloves garlic, minced
1 tsp. dried oregano
½ tsp. creole seasoning
freshly ground black pepper to taste
1 recipe of Garlic Toast (pg. 126)

Mix together all ingredients but garlic toast in a large bowl; cover and refrigerate 1 hour.

Equally divide and place a mound of salad on each serving plate with 1 slice hot garlic toast alongside.

Serves 4.

Per Serving: 121 Calories

Protein 4 gr.	Carb. 24 gr.
Fat 1 gr.	Cal. from fat 11%
Chol. 0 mg.	Sodium 310 mg.

dinners

FORTY-THREE MEALS

Steam Savory Vegetables

Vegetables cooked to the point of mushiness require a lot of seasoning to give them any taste at all, which creates the need some people have for bacon grease and lard.

But steaming vegetables to a crisp tender stage allows the full flavor to be present in the vegetable, and the use of herbs and spices complements the fresh taste. Adding a garlic clove or onion slice to the steaming water or stock increases the flavor even more.

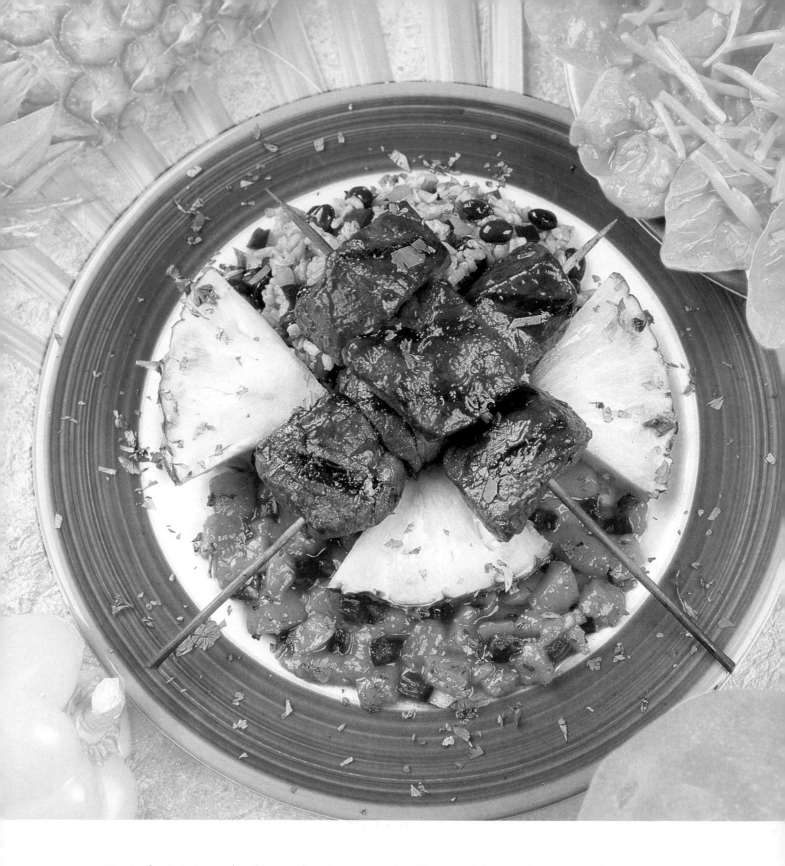

Fruit, fruit juices, herbs and spices are the flavor ribbons that wind through this meal from the tropics. The meat is marinated for tenderness and zest, then placed on a vibrant salsa of mango and red pepper. A bowlful of Caribbean rice and beans makes the perfect accompaniment.

A Taste of the Tropics

beef, black beans (protein)
rice, black beans (complex carb.)
mango, spinach (simple carb.)

Beef Tip Skewers

1 ½ lbs. beef sirloin, cut into chunks
¾ cup Balsamic Marinade (pg. 56)
12 wooden skewers
1 tsp. creole seasoning
½ cup Pickapeppa sauce
    (or hot pepper sauce)
2 cups Mango Salsa (pg. 130)
6 pineapple slices
3 Tbsp. tomato, finely chopped
3 Tbsp. chopped fresh parsley

Trim all visible fat from beef. In a large bowl, marinate sirloin chunks in Balsamic Marinade for at least 3 hours; skewer evenly onto wooden skewers that have been soaked in water. Sprinkle with seasoning and grill, brushing with Pickapeppa sauce to coat.

Grill about 4 minutes on one side; turn and grill another 4 minutes or until desired doneness. Spoon ⅓ cup Mango Salsa on each plate. Top with beef skewers, 2 per serving.

Cut each pineapple slice into 3 triangles; arrange around beef tips. Sprinkle with tomatoes and chopped parsley.

Serves 6.

Per Serving: 245 Calories

Protein 27 gr.	Carb. 22 gr.
Fat 9 gr.	Cal. from fat 36%
Chol. 76 mg.	Sodium 718 mg.

Rice and Black Beans

1 tsp. olive oil
½ red onion, diced
2 cloves garlic, minced
1 cup chicken stock (fat-free/low salt)
1 ½ cups tomato sauce
1 cup long-grain brown rice, uncooked
½ cup black beans, drained
    and rinsed
½ tsp. cumin
½ tsp. creole seasoning

Spray saucepan with cooking spray; add olive oil and heat. Add diced onion and garlic, and sauté. Add chicken stock and tomato sauce. When boiling, add rice. Simmer for 1 minute; then cover and steam until done, about 40 to 45 minutes.

Combine black beans with cumin and seasoning. Microwave 1 ½ minutes on high. Using a large slotted spoon, smash beans until half are mush. Combine with hot, cooked rice.

Serves 6.

Per Serving: 161 Calories

Protein 4 gr.	Carb. 33 gr.
Fat 1 gr.	Cal. from fat 6%
Chol. 0 mg.	Sodium 460 mg.

(Meal continued on the next page)

A Taste of the Tropics (continued)

Tropical Spinach Salad

12 oz. fresh spinach, washed and stemmed
3 navel oranges, peeled and sectioned
1 whole carrot, cut lengthwise into strips
1 cup Honey-Orange Vinaigrette
2 tomatoes, diced fine
2 Tbsp. dry-roasted pistachios, shelled

Toss spinach, orange sections and carrot strips with Honey-Orange Vinaigrette. Sprinkle with diced tomato and pistachios.
Serves 4.

Per Serving: 138 Calories

Protein 4 gr.	Carb. 26 gr.
Fat 2 gr.	Cal. from fat 13%
Chol. 0 mg.	Sodium 184 mg.

Honey-Orange Vinaigrette

½ cup orange juice
1 Tbsp. honey
½ cup balsamic vinegar
½ tsp. creole seasoning
1 tsp. Pickapeppa sauce (or hot pepper sauce)
juice of ½ lemon
1 Tbsp. chopped fresh herbs (cilantro, basil, rosemary, thyme)

Mix together all ingredients. Refrigerate.
Makes 10 servings, 2 Tbsp. each.

Per Serving: 12 Calories

Protein 0 gr.	Carb. 3 gr.
Fat 0 gr.	Cal. from fat 0%
Chol. 0 mg.	Sodium 53 mg.

Mango Salsa

2 whole ripe mangos, peeled and diced
juice of 2 limes
½ cup orange juice
1 large red bell pepper, diced
½ tsp. five spice powder
½ Tbsp. minced shallots, diced fine
¼ cup honey
1 tsp. creole seasoning

Mix together all ingredients. Refrigerate at least 1 hour to blend flavors.
Makes 8 servings, ⅓ cup each.

Per Serving: 77 Calories

Protein 0 gr.	Carb. 20 gr.
Fat 0 gr.	Cal. from fat 0
Chol. 0 mg.	Sodium 135 mg.

Super Supper Burger

turkey (protein)
bread (complex carb.)
tomato, cucumbers (simple carb.)

Super Supper Burger

1½ lbs. ground turkey breast
1 small green bell pepper, chopped
1 small onion, minced
1 Tbsp. grated horseradish
1 Tbsp. Dijon mustard
1 tsp. creole seasoning
¼ cup chili sauce (or salsa)*
1 round unsliced Italian loaf or
   sourdough bread, 8 inches in diameter, preferably whole wheat
2 large leaves of lettuce

* either one can be purchased in any
   grocery store

Preheat oven to 350 degrees.

In a large bowl, mix all ingredients except chili sauce, bread and lettuce. Press meat mixture into an ungreased 9-inch pie plate. Spread chili sauce on top.

Bake uncovered 45 minutes or until meat is no longer pink in the center. Drain immediately upon removing from oven. Let stand 5 minutes. Cut bread crosswise into halves (like a large bun). Carefully place pie-size burger on one bread half. Top with lettuce and other half of bread. Cut into six wedges.

Serves 6.

Per Serving: 259 Calories

Protein 28 gr.	Carb. 26 gr.
Fat 5 gr.	Cal. from fat 17%
Chol. 52 mg.	Sodium 712 mg.

Spicy Tomato and Cucumber Salad

2 large tomatoes, cut into wedges
1 cup diced cucumber
½ cup finely chopped red onion
1 clove garlic, minced
2 Tbsp. chopped fresh cilantro
2 Tbsp. red wine vinegar
2 tsp. chopped fresh hot green chili
   pepper (or ¼ tsp. crushed red pepper)
1 tsp. honey
½ tsp. creole seasoning

In a medium-sized bowl, mix together all ingredients. Cover and refrigerate about 2 hours or until chilled.

Makes 6 servings.

Per Serving: 28 Calories

Protein 1 gr.	Carb. 6 gr.
Fat 0 gr.	Cal. from fat 0%
Chol. 0 mg.	Sodium 96 mg.

Tips for Tomato Lovers

Ripen tomatoes with an apple in a paper bag pierced with a few holes. Once ripened, store tomatoes, stem down, at room temperature away from direct sunlight. Never refrigerate tomatoes! Cold temperatures make the flesh pulpy and destroy the flavor.

If you are using canned tomatoes in a recipe, go for canned Italian plum tomatoes—they have a wonderful flavor that sometimes even beats fresh, out-of-season tomatoes.

Masterful Meatloaf

meat (protein)
oats, potatoes (complex carb.)
tomatoes, broccoli (simple carb.)

Masterful Meatloaf

2 lbs. ground round (or ground turkey breast)
¾ cup chopped onion
2 cloves garlic, minced
2 cups old-fashioned oats, uncooked
2 Tbsp. tomato purée
2 tsp. Dijon mustard
1 tsp. creole seasoning
1 Tbsp. Worcestershire sauce
2 egg whites (or ¼ cup egg substitute)
2 Tbsp. skim milk
½ cup tomato sauce (or salsa)

Preheat oven to 375 degrees.

Spray two loaf pans with cooking spray. Mix together all ingredients except tomato sauce; shape into 2 loaves and place in loaf pans.

Bake about 1 hour or until no longer pink in center. Drain off all juices immediately upon removing from oven. One loaf may be frozen for a later meal.

Spread with even amounts of tomato sauce or salsa. Cut each loaf into 6 slices.

One loaf makes 6 servings, 1 slice per serving.

Per Serving: 175 Calories

Protein 24 gr.	Carb. 13 gr.
Fat 3 gr.	Cal. from fat 17%
Chol. 47 mg.	Sodium 278 mg.

Oven Potato Casserole

4 cups thinly sliced Idaho potatoes
1 red onion, sliced thin
2 large tomatoes, sliced thin
1 tsp. creole seasoning
½ cup part-skim cheddar cheese, shredded

Preheat oven to 350 degrees.

Alternate layers of potatoes, onions and tomatoes in baking dish. Lightly sprinkle each layer with seasoning.

Bake for 30 minutes (or microwave on high for 12 minutes). Top with cheese in the last 5 minutes of cooking and allow to melt, gently browning.

Makes 6 servings.

Per Serving: 99 Calories

Protein 4 gr.	Carb. 18 gr.
Fat 1.5 gr.	Cal. from fat 15%
Chol. 5 mg.	Sodium 229 mg.

Seasoned Broccoli

1½ lbs. fresh broccoli, trimmed
⅓ cup chicken stock (fat-free/low salt)
1 tsp. Mrs. Dash seasoning
¾ tsp. creole seasoning

Microwave broccoli in chicken stock and seasonings for 7 to 8 minutes or until crisp tender. Serves 6.

Per Serving: 48 Calories

Protein 4 gr.	Carb. 8 gr.
Fat 0 gr.	Cal. from fat 0%
Chol. 0 mg.	Sodium 168 mg.

Savory Round Roast

roast (protein)
polenta (complex carb.)
green beans (simple carb.)

Savory Round Roast

1 boneless round roast (about 4 lbs.),
   trimmed of all fat
1 tsp. ground ginger
1 tsp. creole seasoning
1 tsp. Mrs. Dash garlic herb seasoning
1 Tbsp. chopped fresh basil (or 1 tsp.
   dried)
2 cloves garlic, minced
2 medium chopped onions
1 cup tomato purée
1 cup dry red wine*

* or substitute dealcoholized wine or
  defatted beef stock (fat-free/low salt)

• **Serve with Green Beans and
Mushrooms (pg. 179).**

Preheat oven to 325 degrees.
Spray nonstick skillet with cooking spray; heat. Brown roast on both sides in skillet. Transfer to a rack in a roasting pan and season with ginger, seasonings and basil.

Add garlic and onions to tomato purée and spread over the top of roast. Slowly pour wine over the top.

Cover tightly and bake for 2½ to 3 hours or until meat is tender, basting several times.

Makes 16 servings. Remaining servings may be frozen in plastic freezer bags for later meals.

Per Serving: 202 Calories

Protein 26 gr.	Carb. 3 gr.
Fat 8 gr.	Cal. from fat 40%
Chol. 76 mg.	Sodium 250 mg.

Polenta Wedges

4 cups water
1 cup frozen whole kernel corn, thawed
   (or 2 ears fresh corn, cooked)
1 tsp. creole seasoning
1 tsp. olive oil
1 Tbsp. fresh whole rosemary (or 1
   tsp. dried)
1 cup stone-ground cornmeal (or
   polenta)

Spray a 9- x 13-inch rectangular baking pan with cooking spray.

In a medium saucepan, heat all ingredients except cornmeal to boiling. Gradually add cornmeal, stirring constantly. Cook over medium-low heat 8 to 12 minutes, stirring occasionally, until mixture pulls away from sides of saucepan. Pour into baking dish. Cool 15 minutes. Cover and refrigerate 1 hour or until firm. Can be refrigerated up to 3 days.

When ready to serve, cut polenta into six squares; cut each square diagonally into 2 triangles. Spray a large nonstick skillet with cooking spray and heat over medium heat. Brown triangles in skillet for about 5 minutes on each side or until light brown.

Serves 6.

Per Serving: 55 Calories

Protein 1 gr.	Carb. 11 gr.
Fat 1 gr.	Cal. from fat 18%
Chol. 0 mg.	Sodium 182 mg.

Polenta or Stone-Ground Cornmeal

Polenta is made from coarse ground cornmeal. It may be used as a grain side dish or in desserts. Polenta can be found in health food stores.

Most cornmeal in supermarkets is steel-ground, which means the husk and germ have been almost completely removed.

Stone-ground cornmeal retains some of the corn's hull and germ, making it more nutritious. To make polenta without lumps, whisk the cornmeal into the cold liquid before heating and cooking.

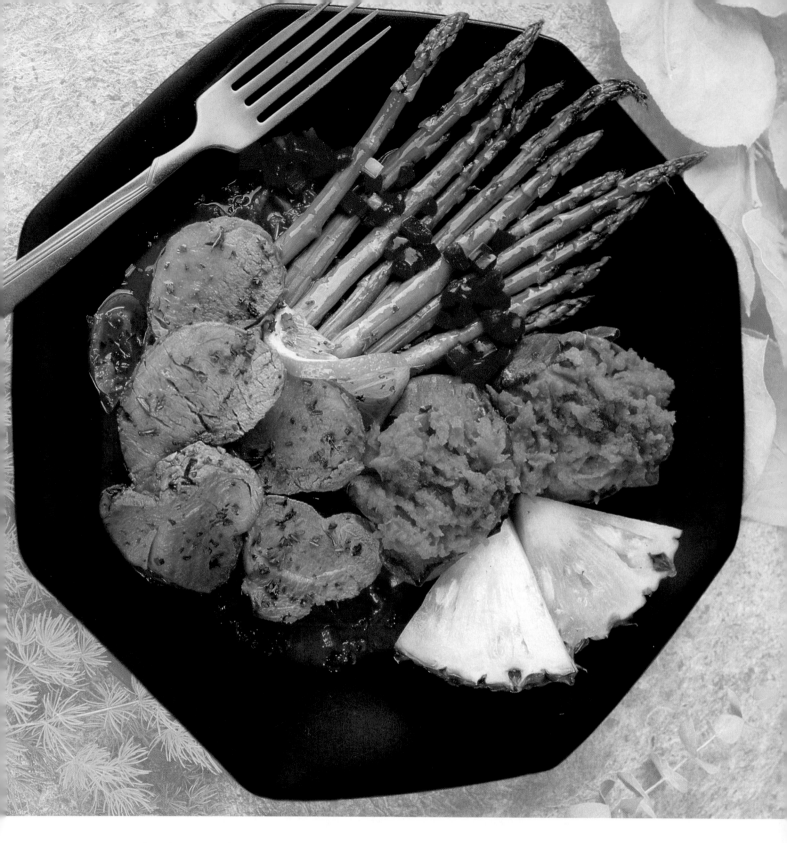

This beautiful menu is a perfect match for any special occasion. It is elegant in presentation, yet simple and quick in preparation. The marinated, seared pork tenderloin goes perfectly with fluffy cinnamon-scented sweet potatoes. And asparagus is the vegetable that heralds freshness.

Speedy Pork Roast

pork (protein)
sweet potatoes (complex carb.)
asparagus (simple carb.)

Seared Pork Tenderloin

1 ½ lbs. pork tenderloin, trimmed of all visible fat
½ cup Lea and Perrins Worcestershire for Chicken
½ tsp. creole seasoning
1 tsp. Mrs. Dash seasoning
2 Tbsp. chopped fresh herbs (cilantro, basil, rosemary, thyme)
2 garlic cloves, minced
1 large red onion, sliced thin

Preheat oven to 400 degrees.
Marinate pork tenderloin in Worcestershire sauce, seasonings, herbs and garlic for at least 1 hour.
Sear pork on both sides in hot ovenproof skillet, then top with sliced onion. Place whole skillet in oven for 15 minutes or until internal temperature reaches 150 to 170 degrees. May pour on additional marinade while roasting.
Serves 4.

Per Serving: 148 Calories

Protein 25 gr.	Carb. 1 gr.
Fat 4 gr.	Cal. from fat 26%
Chol. 78 mg.	Sodium 190 mg.

Cinnamon Sweet Potatoes

4 sweet potatoes
cinnamon

Preheat oven to 400 degrees.
Wash and scrub sweet potatoes. Place in oven for 35 minutes. (You may add the skillet of pork tenderloins to the oven after 20 minutes.)
Cut open sweet potatoes and push ends together to "mash" toward center and fluff. Sprinkle with cinnamon.
Serves 4.

Per Serving: 118 Calories

Protein 2 gr.	Carb. 27 gr.
Fat 0 gr.	Cal. from fat 0%
Chol. 0 mg.	Sodium 12 mg.

Fresh Asparagus

1 lb. fresh asparagus, trimmed
¼ cup chicken stock (fat-free/low salt)
1 tsp. Mrs. Dash seasoning
½ tsp. creole seasoning

Microwave asparagus in chicken stock and seasonings for about 7 to 8 minutes or until crisp tender.
Serves 4.

Per Serving: 48 Calories

Protein 4 gr.	Carb. 8 gr.
Fat 0 gr.	Cal. from fat 0%
Chol. 0 mg.	Sodium 140 mg.

Cooking Temperatures for Meat

Cooking pork to 137 degrees will kill trichinosis. To allow for a safety margin, however, most experts recommend an internal temperature of 150 to 165 degrees. This range will produce pork that's juicy and tender. Pork cooked to temperatures above 170 degrees will be dry and overcooked. Use a meat thermometer (purchased at the supermarket or department store's kitchen section) to check for doneness.

Pork Chops Portofino

pork chops, cheese (protein)
bread crumbs, orzo (complex carb.)
broccoli, grapes (simple carb.)

**Fat-Free Flavor:
Sun-Dried Tomatoes**

*Use sun-dried tomatoes
for added depth of fla-
vor without the fat; their
dark red color and crin-
kled flesh are an espe-
cially welcome boost to
sauces.*

*Buy sun-dried tomatoes
packaged in plastic;
soak back to life in boiling water for 2 minutes,
then drain.*

Pork Chops Portofino

½ cup feta cheese
¼ cup skim-milk ricotta cheese
2 Tbsp. sun-dried tomatoes, slivered
⅛ tsp. cracked black pepper
1 Tbsp. fresh Italian parsley (or parsley)
1 tsp. Mrs. Dash seasoning
4 center-cut pork chops
    (about 1¼ lbs.), trimmed of fat
2 large egg whites
¼ cup water
⅔ cup dried Italian bread crumbs
    (purchased)
2 Tbsp. grated Parmesan cheese
½ tsp. creole seasoning

• Serve with 2 cups cooked orzo and
  a side of Frosted Grapes (pg. 140)

Preheat oven to 400 degrees.
Mix together cheeses, tomatoes, pepper, parsley and Mrs. Dash to make stuffing; set aside.

Place the pork chops on a cutting board. With
a sharp knife, make a horizontal slit along the
long edge of each chop opposite the bone,
nearly cutting through to the opposite side.
Open the chop so it forms a butterfly. Place one-
fourth of the cheese mixture on half of each
chop, leaving a ¼-inch space between the filling and the edges of the meat. Close the chop
carefully and set aside. Repeat with the remaining pork chops.

Whisk together egg whites and water in a
bowl. In a shallow pan, stir together bread
crumbs, Parmesan cheese and creole seasoning.

Spray a shallow roasting pan with cooking
spray. Carefully dip each chop in the crumb mixture, then in the egg white mixture and back
again in the crumb mixture. Gently lift into the
baking pan and bake for 40 to 45 minutes, until
crisp and lightly browned on the outside and

juices run clear.
Serves 4.

Per Serving: 274 Calories

Protein 32 gr.	Carb. 15 gr.
Fat 8 gr.	Cal. from fat 26%
Chol. 93 mg.	Sodium 535 mg.

Tuscan Broccoli

1 tsp. olive oil
2 cloves garlic, minced
2 Tbsp. capers, rinsed
½ tsp. creole seasoning
1 tsp. Mrs. Dash seasoning
1 Tbsp. chopped fresh rosemary (or
    1 tsp. dried)
1 bunch (1¼ lbs.) broccoli, cut into
    florets and trimmed of tough stalks
½ cup chicken stock (fat-free/low salt)

Spray a large nonstick skillet with cooking
spray. Add olive oil and heat over medium heat.
Add garlic, capers, seasonings and rosemary,
and sauté until the garlic is golden, about 30
seconds. Add the broccoli florets and chicken
stock. Reduce heat and cook covered until broccoli is crisp tender and cooking liquid is reduced,
about 5 to 7 minutes. Ladle into serving dish,
tossing together.
Serves 4.

Per Serving: 57 Calories

Protein 4 gr.	Carb. 8 gr.
Fat 1 gr.	Cal. from fat 16%
Chol. 0 mg.	Sodium 688 mg.

Marinated Pork Tenderloin

pork (protein)
black beans, rice (complex carb.)
vegetables (simple carb.)

Marinated Pork Tenderloin

¼ cup low-sodium soy sauce
2 Tbsp. ginger
2 cups red wine*
¼ cup Dijon mustard
2 Tbsp. chopped fresh basil
juice of 1 lemon
1½ lbs. pork tenderloin, trimmed of fat
1 carrot, quartered
1 cup green beans, trimmed
1 small red onion, chopped
4 shiitake mushrooms (optional)
2 Tbsp. chopped fresh herbs (cilantro,
     basil, rosemary, thyme)
1 tsp. creole seasoning
2 tsp. Mrs. Dash seasoning

* or substitute dealcoholized wine or
  chicken stock (fat-free/low salt)

● Serve with Rice and Black Beans (pg.
  129).

Mix soy, ginger, wine, mustard, basil and lemon juice for marinade. Marinate pork overnight.
Preheat oven to 400 degrees.
In a microwaveable dish, place carrots, green beans, onion and mushrooms with ½ cup water. Cover with plastic wrap and vent. Microwave on high for 4 to 5 minutes.
Spray a nonstick ovenproof skillet with cooking spray; heat over medium-high heat. Add the marinated tenderloin (reserve remaining marinade) and sear on both sides.
Transfer skillet to oven; cook to medium pink or an internal temperature of 150 to 170 degrees.
Remove pork from pan. In same pan, sauté the vegetables with fresh herbs and seasonings.

Add pork. Add 2 Tbsp. of reserved pork marinade; cook for 3 to 4 minutes.
  Serves 4.

Per Serving: 201 Calories

Protein 27 gr.	Carb. 13 gr.
Fat 4 gr.	Cal. from fat 18%
Chol. 79 mg.	Sodium 725 mg.

Fresh Vegetables With Creamy Herb Dip

2 oz. fat-free cream cheese, softened
2 Tbsp. nonfat sour cream
2 Tbsp. chopped fresh chives (or scallions)
1 Tbsp. chopped fresh dill
½ tsp. creole seasoning
1 tsp. Mrs. Dash seasoning
1 tsp. prepared horseradish
2 cups trimmed and sliced fresh vegetables (carrots, broccoli, cucumbers, celery, zucchini, yellow squash, red and green bell pepper strips)

Place cream cheese in a small bowl and stir in nonfat sour cream until smooth. Mix in chives, dill, seasonings and horseradish. Spoon into small bowl. Surround bowl with vegetables.
  Serves 4.

Per Serving: 26 Calories

Protein 3.5 gr.	Carb. 3 gr.
Fat 0 gr.	Cal. from fat 0%
Chol. 1 mg.	Sodium 208 mg.

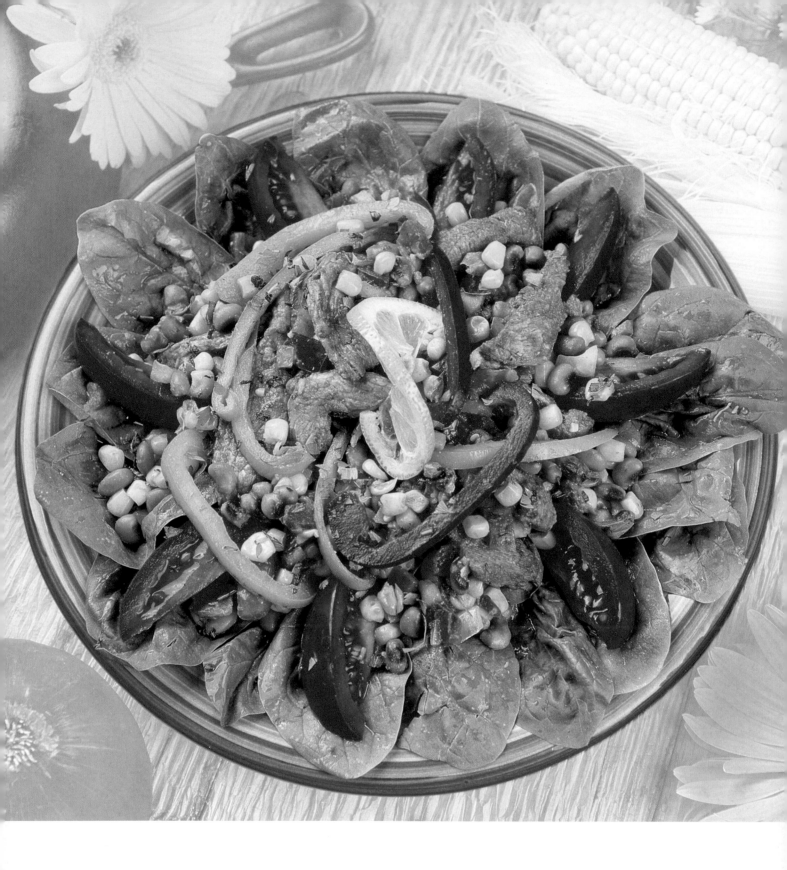

A dish of pork and black-eyed peas is soul food in the South—the original comfort food. Lean and tender pork is marinated in Balsamic Marinade, then seared. Combined with the black-eyed peas and spinach, it becomes a new version of the time-tested favorite.

Southern Pork Salad

pork (protein)
black-eyed peas, corn (complex carb.)
spinach, peppers (simple carb.)

Seared Pork and Black-Eyed Pea Salad

1 lb. pork tenderloin or medallions, cut into strips
½ cup Balsamic Marinade (pg. 56)
2 cloves garlic, minced
1 each red and green bell peppers, quartered
2 cups Black-Eyed Pea and Corn Salad
12 oz. fresh spinach, washed and stemmed
1 Tbsp. chopped fresh herbs (cilantro, basil, rosemary, thyme)
2 plum tomatoes, quartered

Marinate pork strips in ¼ cup Balsamic Marinade for up to 1 hour.

Spray a nonstick skillet with cooking spray. Add garlic and lightly sauté. Add pork to skillet, sautéing 2 to 3 minutes until no pink remains. Add remaining marinade, peppers and Black-Eyed Pea and Corn Salad to skillet, lightly tossing to heat.

Line plate with spinach; top with pork salad mixture, allowing peppers to lie on top. Garnish with herbs and tomato quarters.

Serves 4.

Per Serving: 304 Calories

Protein 32 gr.	Carb. 31 gr.
Fat 7 gr.	Cal. from fat 21%
Chol. 78 mg.	Sodium 332 mg.

Black-Eyed Pea and Corn Salad

16 oz. (or 2 cups frozen) black-eyed peas
¼ cup chicken stock (fat-free/low salt)
1 cup frozen corn kernels, thawed
2 plum tomatoes, diced
¾ red onion, minced
1 serrano pepper, minced
2 Tbsp. finely chopped cilantro
1 tsp. olive oil
4 cloves garlic, minced
juice of 1 lime
¼ cup Balsamic Marinade (pg. 56)
1 tsp. cumin
2 tsp. hot pepper sauce
1 tsp. creole seasoning

Follow package instructions to cook black-eyed peas in ¼ cup chicken stock; cool. Combine all ingredients. Allow to marinate at least one hour.

Makes 8 servings, ½ cup per serving.

Per Serving: 85 Calories

Protein 4 gr.	Carb. 15 gr.
Fat 1 gr.	Cal. from fat 10%
Chol. 0 mg.	Sodium 170 mg.

Precautions for Pork

Just as the commercials say, today's pork is leaner—some cuts are even leaner than beef. And, thanks to modern technology, trichinosis in pork is no longer an issue. Take precautions, however, by thoroughly washing in hot, soapy water anything (hands, knives, cutting boards, etc.) that comes in contact with raw pork. Never taste uncooked pork. Leftover pork dishes should be refrigerated within 2 hours of cooking and used within 2 days.

Grilled Citrus BBQ Pork Chops

pork chops (protein)
plantains (complex carb.)
spinach, grapes (simple carb.)

Citrus BBQ Pork Chops

4 pork chops (7 oz. each) with bone
   (or 1 ½ lbs. center-cut pork chops)
½ cup Jamaican Marinade (pg. 57)
¼ cup Citrus BBQ Sauce (pg. 56)
1 tsp. olive oil
1 small onion, sliced thin
2 cloves garlic, minced
1 ripe plantain, sliced thin
1 cup orange juice
½ tsp. five spice powder (or cinnamon)
1 Tbsp. honey

Trim pork chops of all fat. Marinate pork
chops in Jamaican Marinade for 3 to 4 hours.
Grill, basting with Citrus BBQ Sauce.

While pork chops are grilling, spray a nonstick
pan with cooking spray; add olive oil and heat.
Add onion, garlic and plantain, and sauté with
orange juice, five spice powder and honey until
it begins to caramelize (make a syrup). Serve
the chops with plantains.

Serves 4.

Per Serving: 276 Calories

Protein 26 gr.	Carb. 30 gr.
Fat 5.5 gr.	Cal. from fat 19%
Chol. 78 mg.	Sodium 326 mg.

Sautéed Spinach

1 tsp. olive oil
2 cloves garlic, minced
1 lb. fresh spinach, washed and
   stemmed
½ tsp. creole seasoning
juice of 1 lemon
1 Tbsp. low-sodium soy sauce

Spray a nonstick skillet with cooking spray;
add oil and heat over medium-high heat. Add
garlic and stir until golden, about 30 seconds.
Add spinach and toss until just wilted, 2 to 4
minutes. Add seasoning, lemon juice and soy
sauce; toss to blend. Serve immediately.

Serves 4.

Per Serving: 41 Calories

Protein 3.5 gr.	Carb. 4.5 gr.
Fat 1 gr.	Cal. from fat 22%
Chol. 0 mg.	Sodium 351 mg.

Frosted Grapes

1 lb. red and/or green grapes, stemmed

Wash grapes and pat dry. Place on a pan in
freezer for 45 minutes. Remove from freezer
and let sit for 2 minutes before serving.

Makes 8 servings, about 12 grapes each.

Per Serving: 40 Calories

Protein 0 gr.	Carb. 10 gr.
Fat 0 gr.	Cal. from fat 0%
Chol. 0 mg.	Sodium 1 mg.

Grilled Lamb Chops and Couscous

lamb (protein)
couscous (complex carb.)
vegetables (simple carb.)

Grilled Lamb Chops and Couscous

4 lamb chops (5 oz. each)
³/₄ cup Balsamic Marinade (pg. 56)
¹/₂ cup quick couscous (purchased)
2 cups chicken stock (fat-free/low salt)
2 Tbsp. chopped fresh herbs (cilantro, basil, rosemary, thyme)
1 tsp. Mrs. Dash seasoning
1 tsp. creole seasoning
¹/₂ eggplant, sliced
1 small zucchini, sliced
1 small yellow squash, sliced
1 red bell pepper, quartered
1 tsp. olive oil
¹/₂ medium onion, minced
2 cloves garlic, minced
2 Tbsp. sliced mushroom
2 cups broccoli florets, blanched
2 cups beef stock (fat-free/low salt)
1 tsp. cracked black pepper
1 Tbsp. chopped fresh basil
1 Tbsp. chopped fresh oregano

Trim all fat from lamb chops. Marinate at least 3 hours in ¹/₂ cup Balsamic Marinade.

Cook couscous according to package directions with chicken stock, herbs and seasonings.

Marinate eggplant, zucchini, squash and bell pepper in ¹/₄ cup marinade. Grill (or roast in 400-degree oven until slightly charred), then dice.

Spray skillet with cooking spray. Add oil and heat. Sauté onions and garlic. Add mushrooms, broccoli and grilled vegetables; quickly sauté. Add beef stock, black pepper, herbs and cooked couscous; quickly sauté, leaving dish moist.

Grill marinated lamb chop (or sear in a hot skillet). Serve over vegetable couscous mixture.

Serves 4.

Per Serving: 248 Calories

Protein 21 gr.	Carb. 22 gr.
Fat 8 gr.	Cal. from fat 29%
Chol. 52 mg.	Sodium 198 mg.

Sliced Fennel and Asparagus Salad

1 whole fennel bulb
10 to 12 asparagus spears
2 tsp. olive oil
juice of 1 lemon
¹/₂ tsp. creole seasoning
1 tsp. Mrs. Dash seasoning
1 small tomato, diced

Trim base from fennel bulb. Remove and discard the fennel stalks and any discolored parts from the bulb. Stand the bulb upright and cut vertically into very thin slices.

Slice asparagus into 2-inch pieces. Place in microwaveable bowl with ¹/₄ cup water; microwave on high for 2 to 3 minutes or until crisp tender. Immerse in ice water bath to chill quickly.

In a small bowl, whisk together the oil, lemon juice and seasonings. Add the sliced fennel, asparagus and diced tomato.

Serves 4.

Per Serving: 86 Calories

Protein 3.5 gr.	Carb. 14 gr.
Fat 2.5 gr.	Cal. from fat 26%
Chol. 0 mg.	Sodium 152 mg.

Tips for Cooking Lamb

Removing most of the excess fat from lamb cuts is not only good for your health, but it also reduces any strong lamb flavor some diners don't enjoy.

If lamb is a bit strong for you, even without the fat, try marinating for 2 hours before cooking. This will also tenderize the meat.

Light Seafood Stew

seafood, goat cheese (protein)
bread (complex carb.)
vegetables (simple carb.)

Buying the Best Seafood

The number-one rule for buying seafood is this: Be choosy when you shop! Seafood may not have seen its ocean home for 8 days, yet it still may be legally labeled as "fresh."

Fresh fish should be resting on top of ice in a case kept at lower than 33 degrees. Cuts of fish should hold together well and be unblemished and shiny. Fish should not be spongy to the touch or smelly to the nose!

Light Seafood Stew

4 small potatoes, medium diced
½ cup diced onion
½ cup diced celery
6 cups chicken stock (fat-free/low salt)
1 cup frozen green peas, thawed
½ cup Spanish sherry or white wine*
2 tsp. saffron
1 tsp. creole seasoning
2 tsp. Mrs. Dash seasoning
2 Tbsp. chopped fresh herbs (cilantro, basil, rosemary, thyme)
1 tsp. Tabasco
2 tsp. Worcestershire sauce
20 mussels, washed
20 clams, washed
2 lbs. any fresh fish
⅓ cup chopped chives

* or substitute dealcoholized wine or more chicken stock

Steam potatoes, onion and celery; add to chicken stock. Add peas, sherry, saffron, seasonings, herbs, Tabasco and Worcestershire sauces. Add mussels and clams, and cook until opened.

Add fish and poach in stock lightly. Ladle into soup bowls. Sprinkle with chives.

Makes 10 servings, 1½ cups each.

Per Serving: 243 Calories

Protein 36 gr.   Carb. 13 gr.
Fat 3.5 gr.   Cal. from fat 14%
Chol. 75 mg.   Sodium 384 mg.

Baguette With Warm Goat Cheese

6 oz. goat cheese
2 Tbsp. chopped fresh herbs (cilantro, basil, rosemary, thyme)
¼ tsp. creole seasoning
juice of ½ lemon
2 large tomatoes, sliced
¼ cup bread crumbs (purchased)
1 baguette (a long narrow loaf of French bread)
¼ cup Balsamic Marinade (pg. 56)
1 cup Tomato Basil Sauce (pg. 59)

Preheat oven to 375 degrees.

Mix goat cheese with herbs, seasoning and lemon juice. Place tomato slices on pan. Top each with 2 Tbsp. goat cheese mixture; sprinkle with 1 Tbsp. bread crumbs and brown in oven.

Slice baguette diagonally into 12 pieces. Dip each slice into Balsamic Marinade; toast under broiler until golden brown. Lay slices beside tomatoes, with warm Tomato Basil Sauce for dipping.

Makes 6 servings, 2 pieces of bread and 2 slices of tomato each.

Per Serving: 193 Calories

Protein 7 gr.   Carb. 30 gr.
Fat 5 gr.   Cal. from fat 23%
Chol. 15 mg.   Sodium 426 mg.

Pasta Shrimp Pomodoro

shrimp (protein)
pasta (complex carb.)
vegetables, salad (simple carb.)

Pasta Shrimp Pomodoro

1 ½ lbs. shrimp, peeled and deveined
¼ cup Lea and Perrins Worcestershire for Chicken
8 oz. dry angel hair pasta
2 cloves garlic, minced
1 small red onion, chopped
2 tsp. olive oil
1 each yellow, orange and red bell peppers, cut into strips
1 tsp. Mrs. Dash seasoning
1 tsp. creole seasoning
1 tsp. dried oregano
½ tsp. dried basil
1 can (32 oz.) whole tomatoes
2 Tbsp. grated Parmesan cheese

Marinate shrimp in Worcestershire sauce for at least 15 minutes.

In a large saucepan, cook pasta in salted water until done. Drain.

Spray a nonstick skillet with cooking spray. Lightly sauté half of the garlic and half of the onion. Add shrimp and sear on one side for 1 minute; then turn and sear on other side.

Spray another skillet with cooking spray and add olive oil; heat. Add remaining garlic and onion; sauté. Then add peppers, seasonings and herbs. Allow peppers to soften, then add tomatoes, breaking up tomatoes with spatula while heating. Allow to simmer and reduce for about 4 to 5 more minutes. Add shrimp, stirring all together. Sprinkle with Parmesan cheese. Serve over cooked pasta.

Serves 4.

Per Serving: 394 Calories

Protein 30 gr.	Carb. 54 gr.
Fat 6 gr.	Cal. from fat 16%
Chol. 225 mg.	Sodium 540 mg.

Salad of Field Greens

4 radicchio leaves
1 cup arugula or watercress, washed
1 head endive, sliced
½ cup Green Goddess Dressing (pg. 52)
2 plum tomatoes, seeded and diced
1 cucumber, peeled, seeded and sliced

Cut radicchio leaves in half. Place on plate. Toss arugula and endive in dressing. Mound on top of radicchio. Sprinkle with tomato and cucumber.

Serves 4.

Per Serving: 40 Calories

Protein 3 gr.	Carb. 7 gr.
Fat 0 gr.	Cal. from fat 0%
Chol. 1 mg.	Sodium 70 mg.

Preparing Perfect Pasta

To cook pasta, use 4 quarts of water per pound of pasta.

Have the water boiling rapidly before adding a touch of salt, then pasta. Squeeze lemon into the water to prevent pasta from sticking together.

Perfectly cooked pasta should be al dente—tender, but still firm to the bite. Pasta to be cooked further in another dish should be cooked for one-third less time initially.

Drain pasta well; only rinse if it's to be used in salad.

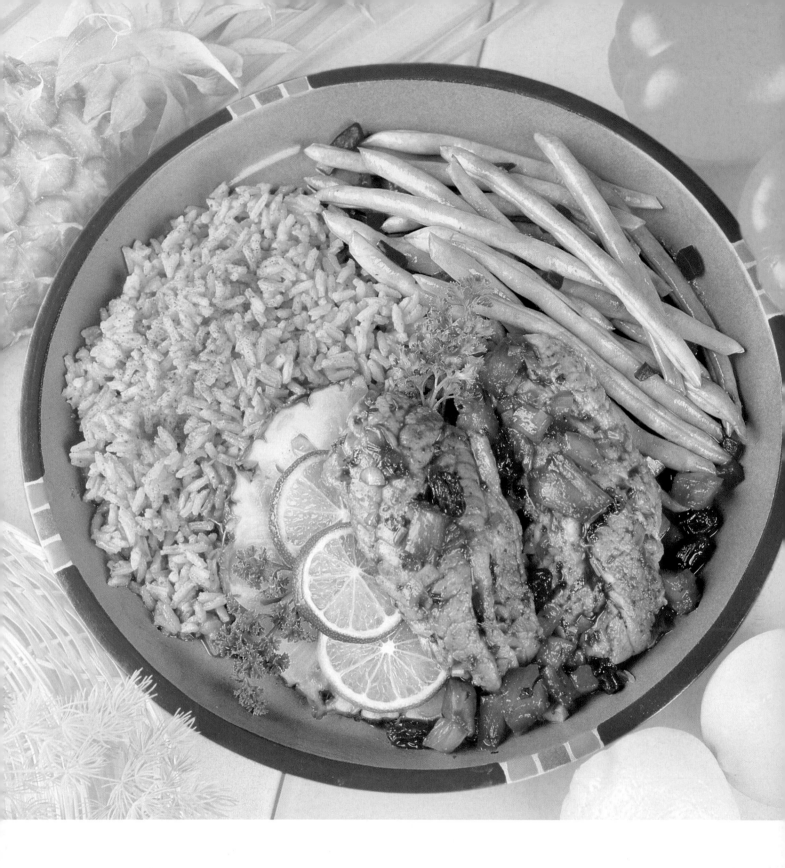

Caribbean cuisine is based on the treasures of the region's soil—extravagantly colored fruits and richly textured vegetables. This cuisine lends itself to cooking the healthy way—fresh and flavorful! This fish is seared with a full-bodied sauce that has an exotic taste of the islands.

Jamaican Grouper

grouper (protein)
rice (complex carb.)
pineapple, raisins, green beans (simple carb.)

Jamaican Grouper

½ cup Lea and Perrins Worcestershire
    for Chicken
4 grouper fillets (5 oz. each)
1 tsp. olive oil
1 tsp. creole seasoning
2 cups Jamaican Sauce
½ cup chicken stock (fat-free/low salt),
    if needed
1 Tbsp. chopped fresh herbs (cilantro,
    basil, rosemary, thyme)

Marinate grouper in Worcestershire sauce.
Spray a nonstick skillet with cooking spray.
Add olive oil and heat. Sprinkle grouper with
seasoning and lightly sear on both sides.
Add Jamaican Sauce to skillet and allow
grouper to finish cooking while sauce is reducing. Add chicken stock, if necessary, to keep
grouper from burning.
Serve grouper with pan sauces. Sprinkle with
herbs.
Serves 4.

Per Serving: 199 Calories

Protein 30 gr.	Carb. 11 gr.
Fat 3 gr.	Cal. from fat 14%
Chol. 53 mg.	Sodium 598 mg.

Jamaican Sauce

1 tsp. olive oil
2 cloves garlic, minced
1 Tbsp. minced shallots
1 tsp. creole seasoning
2 cups beef stock (fat-free/low salt)
¼ diced fresh pineapple (about ½ cup)
2 Tbsp. Jamaican dark rum (optional)
½ tsp. five spice powder
1 Tbsp. honey
2 Tbsp. golden raisins
1 Tbsp. Pickapeppa sauce (or hot
    pepper sauce)
1 Tbsp. chopped fresh herbs (cilantro,
    basil, rosemary, thyme)

Spray a nonstick skillet with cooking spray.
Add olive oil and heat. Sprinkle garlic and shallots with seasoning and quickly sauté 1 to 2
minutes. Add stock and allow to reduce while
adding remaining ingredients. Add extra stock as
needed.
Makes 2 cups, ¼ cup per serving.

Per Serving: 31 Calories

Protein 0 gr.	Carb. 8 gr.
Fat less than 1 gr.	Cal. from fat 0%
Chol. 0 mg.	Sodium 134 mg.

(Meal continued on the next page)

Have You Had Your Fish Oil Today?

All fish contain wonderfully healthy oils that lower total cholesterol while increasing your level of the good HDL cholesterol. Those highest in disease-preventing oils, omega-3's, are cold-water fish and hard shellfish, such as salmon, albacore tuna, swordfish, sardines and mackerel.

These fish oils have also been shown to reduce the tendency of the blood to clot and to decrease triglycerides— and even to help battle arthritis!

So have you had your fish today?

Jamaican Grouper (continued)

Saffron Rice

1 tsp. olive oil
2 cloves garlic, minced
1 3/4 cups chicken stock (fat-free/low salt)
4 to 5 saffron threads (or 1/4 tsp. powder)
1/8 tsp. cumin
1 tsp. creole seasoning
1 Tbsp. chopped fresh parsley (or 1 tsp. dried)
2 cups instant brown rice

Spray a medium saucepan with cooking spray. Add olive oil and heat. Add garlic and lightly sauté about 1 to 2 minutes, then add chicken stock, saffron, cumin, seasoning and herbs. Bring to a boil, then stir in brown rice. Boil for 1 minute; turn heat down to low and cover. Simmer for 5 minutes; uncover saucepan and fluff rice with fork. Cover again and let sit for another 5 minutes.
Serves 4.

Per Serving: 126 Calories

Protein 2.5 gr.	Carb. 24 gr.
Fat 2 gr.	Cal. from fat 15%
Chol. 0 mg.	Sodium 136 mg.

Roasted Green Beans and Peppers

3/4 lb. green beans, trimmed
1 large red bell pepper, cut into long thin strips
1 tsp. olive oil
1/2 tsp. creole seasoning
1 tsp. Mrs. Dash seasoning

Preheat oven to 450 degrees.
Place green beans and pepper strips on a baking sheet and toss with olive oil and seasonings. Spread the vegetables in an even layer. Roast for about 12 minutes or until the vegetables are browned and tender. Stir midway.
Serves 4.

Per Serving: 57 Calories

Protein 2 gr.	Carb. 10 gr.
Fat 1 gr.	Cal. from fat 16%
Chol. 0 mg.	Sodium 140 mg.

Herb-Crusted Orange Roughy

fish (protein)
potatoes, bread crumbs (complex carb.)
broccoli (simple carb.)

Herb-Crusted Orange Roughy

4 orange roughy fillets (5 oz. each)
¼ cup Lea and Perrins Worcestershire for Chicken
1 tsp. creole seasoning
2 Tbsp. chopped fresh herbs (cilantro, basil, rosemary, thyme)
½ cup dried bread crumbs (purchased)
¼ cup Dijon mustard
½ cup Tomato Basil Sauce (pg. 59)
2 cups broccoli florets, steamed until crisp tender
1 Tbsp. parsley, chopped

Marinate orange roughy in Worcestershire sauce for at least 15 minutes, or up to 1 hour.

Preheat oven to 375 degrees.

Season fish with seasoning and herbs, and roll in bread crumbs. Spread mustard on top of fish and roll in bread crumbs once more.

Spray a nonstick skillet with cooking spray; heat. Sear fish in hot skillet on both sides, then transfer to oven and roast until done and browned.

Serve on bed of Tomato Basil Sauce with steamed broccoli. Sprinkle with chopped parsley.

Serves 4.

Per Serving: 291 Calories

Protein 36 gr.	Carb. 29 gr.
Fat 4 gr.	Cal. from fat 14%
Chol. 53 mg.	Sodium 723 mg.

Herb-Roasted Potatoes

2 lbs. (about 5 large) red-skinned potatoes, scrubbed and quartered
2 cloves garlic, minced
2 tsp. olive oil
½ tsp. creole seasoning
1 tsp. Mrs. Dash seasoning
1 Tbsp. chopped fresh rosemary (or 1 tsp. dried)

Preheat oven to 450 degrees.

Spray a shallow roasting pan with cooking spray. Add potatoes, garlic, olive oil, seasonings and rosemary, and spread in an even layer. Bake until the potatoes begin to brown, 20 to 30 minutes, turning them once midway through roasting.

Serves 4.

Per Serving: 139 Calories

Protein 2 gr.	Carb. 27 gr.
Fat 2 gr.	Cal. from fat 15%
Chol. 0 mg.	Sodium 139 mg.

Low-Fat Baked Potato Toppings

A baked potato doesn't have to be piled with butter and sour cream to be delicious. Here are some low-fat suggestions for seasoning these packages of power:

- *Nonfat yogurt, sour cream or blended-till-smooth nonfat cottage cheese (or ricotta) mixed with chopped chives, fresh dill, parsley, scallions, horseradish or minced green pepper*

- *Salsa and herbs*

- *Dried herbs mixed with a little lemon juice or balsamic vinegar*

- *Fresh grated Parmesan cheese*

- *Dijon mustard or low-fat salad dressing*

Curried Shrimp

shrimp (protein)
cornsticks (complex carb.)
vegetables (simple carb.)

Curried Shrimp

1 lb. large shrimp, peeled and
  deveined
½ cup Balsamic Marinade (pg. 56)
1 tsp. curry powder
1 tsp. olive oil
1 small onion, finely chopped
2 cloves garlic, minced
1 tsp. creole seasoning
1 cup white wine*
2 Tbsp. grenadine
¼ cup Lea and Perrins Worcestershire
  for Chicken
1 to 1½ cups chicken stock
  (fat-free/low salt)
3 plum tomatoes, cut into eighths
1 lb. frozen corn kernels, thawed
2 Tbsp. chopped fresh herbs (cilantro,
  basil, rosemary, thyme)
1 lemon

* *or substitute dealcoholized wine or more
  chicken stock*

- Serve with a salad tossed with
  Peppercorn-Parmesan Dressing
  (pg. 53).

Marinate shrimp in Balsamic Marinade for up
to 1 hour. Sprinkle with curry powder.

Spray large nonstick skillet with cooking
spray. Add olive oil and heat. Add onion and garlic, and sauté. Add drained shrimp. Sprinkle with
seasoning. Turn shrimp as it browns.

Add white wine, grenadine and Worcestershire sauce. Add 1 cup chicken stock, tomatoes,
corn and fresh herbs. Reduce liquid by one half,
adding more chicken stock as needed. Squeeze
lemon juice over all.

Serves 4.

Per Serving: 227 Calories

Protein 22 gr.	Carb. 28 gr.
Fat 3 gr.	Cal. from fat 12%
Chol. 166 mg.	Sodium 733 mg.

Cheesy Cornsticks

⅓ cup skim milk
2 egg whites, lightly beaten
1 Tbsp. olive oil
⅓ cup whole-wheat pastry flour
½ cup stone-ground cornmeal
¼ cup grated Parmesan cheese
2 tsp. baking powder
½ tsp. sugar
¼ tsp. salt

Preheat oven to 425 degrees.

Spray a muffin pan or cast-iron cornstick
mold with cooking spray.

Combine milk, egg whites and oil in a measuring cup; stir briskly with a fork until mixed. In a
medium-sized bowl, whisk together flour, cornmeal, cheese, baking powder, sugar and salt.
Make a well in the center of the dry mixture and
pour in the milk mixture. Stir until just combined.

Spoon a heaping tablespoon of the batter
into each of 8 cornstick molds or divide the batter among 4 muffin cups. Bake for 10 to 12
minutes or until set and lightly browned.

Makes 8 cornsticks.

Per Serving: 83 Calories

Protein 4 gr.	Carb. 10 gr.
Fat 3 gr.	Cal. from fat 32%
Chol. 2 mg.	Sodium 231 mg.

Roasted Cod With Vegetables

codfish (protein)
rice, green peas (complex carb.)
vegetables, salad (simple carb.)

Roasted Cod With Vegetables

4 codfish fillets (5 oz. each)
½ cup Balsamic Marinade (pg. 56)
1 large stalk celery, diced
1 red bell pepper, diced
1 carrot, diced
½ cup diced fennel
½ cup diced red onion
1 tsp. creole seasoning
3 cups chicken stock (fat-free/low salt)
½ cup white wine*
2 whole tomatoes, seeded and chopped
1 can (4 oz.) tomato paste
1 tsp. Mrs. Dash seasoning
2 cups green peas

* or substitute dealcoholized wine or more chicken stock

Preheat oven to 350 degrees.

Marinate codfish in Balsamic Marinade. Spray a large, nonstick ovenproof skillet with cooking spray. Sear codfish over medium-high heat on both sides. Then put skillet in oven for 6 to 8 minutes to finish cooking.

Steam celery, bell pepper, carrot and fennel over boiling water, or microwave, covered and vented, on high power with ¼ cup water for 3 to 4 minutes.

Spray another pan with cooking spray; heat. Quickly sauté onions; add creole seasoning and steamed vegetables. Sauté lightly; add chicken stock and wine. Cook and reduce by half.

Add tomatoes and tomato paste; cook for 1 minute. Add Mrs. Dash and cook until vegetables are done. Add green peas. Pour broth and vegetables into bowl; top with codfish.

Serves 4.

Per Serving: 291 Calories

Protein 29 gr.	Carb. 37 gr.
Fat 3 gr.	Cal. from fat 9%
Chol. 35 mg.	Sodium 706 mg.

Crunchy Jicama and Melon Salad

1 medium jicama, julienned
1 medium cantaloupe, cut into ½-inch cubes
3 Tbsp. lime juice
3 Tbsp. chopped fresh mint (or 1 Tbsp. dried)
1 tsp. grated lime peel
2 tsp. honey
¼ tsp. salt

In a medium-sized bowl, mix together all ingredients. Cover and refrigerate 2 hours or until chilled.

Makes 4 servings.

Per Serving: 62 Calories

Protein 1 gr.	Carb. 15 gr.
Fat 0 gr.	Cal. from fat 0%
Chol. 0 mg.	Sodium 91 mg.

What's Jicama?

Jicama is a large root vegetable with a thin brown skin and white crunchy flesh. Its nutty, sweet flavor resembles water chestnuts and is great both raw and cooked. It's good raw added to fruit and vegetable salads. It also adds crunch when sliced thin for sandwiches. Cooked, it can be used in stir-fried dishes. Or it can be boiled and mashed like potatoes, added to soups and stews at the end of their cooking, or just sautéed on its own.

Shop for a jicama that's heavy for its size and free of blemishes. One pound yields about 3 cups chopped. Store jicama in a plastic bag in the refrigerator for up to 2 weeks. Pull off skin with a sharp knife just before using.

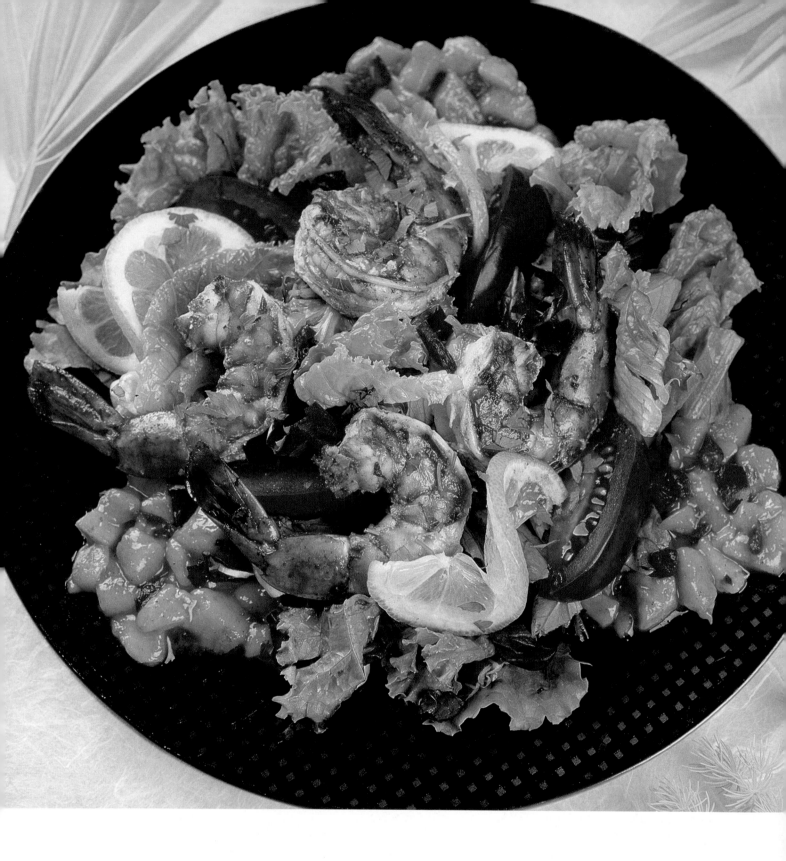

The beauty of this meal is that its preparation does not require a great deal of time: The shrimp is cooked quickly, and the salsa is prepared ahead of time. The focaccia bread accompaniment can either be purchased or prepared in advance, making a perfectly balanced meal.

Shrimp Salad St. Lucia

shrimp (protein)
bread (complex carb.)
salsa, vegetables (simple carb.)

Shrimp Salad St. Lucia

1 ¼ lbs. large shrimp
¼ cup Lea and Perrins Worcestershire for Chicken
1 tsp. olive oil
1 tsp. creole seasoning
1 cup Mango Salsa
8 cups washed, dried and torn mixed greens (red leaf, romaine, frizee, radicchio, arugula or bibb)
½ cup Citrus Vinaigrette (pg. 52)
2 tomatoes, cut into wedges
2 lemons, sliced thin
2 Tbsp. chopped fresh herbs (cilantro, basil, rosemary, thyme)

Serve with Focaccia Bread (pg. 158).

Peel all but tails of shrimp; devein. Marinate shrimp in Worcestershire sauce for at least 1 hour.

Spray a nonstick skillet with cooking spray. Add olive oil and heat. Sprinkle shrimp with seasoning and quickly sauté in hot pan until done.

To serve, spoon 3 small pools of salsa on each plate. Toss torn lettuce leaves with Citrus Vinaigrette. Place lettuce in middle of plate. Then arrange shrimp and tomato wedges on top of salad.

Garnish with lemon slices and sprinkle with chopped herbs.

Serves 4.

Per Serving: 341 Calories

Protein 27 gr.	Carb. 48 gr.
Fat 4.5 gr.	Cal. from fat 12%
Chol. 166 mg.	Sodium 625 mg.

Mango Salsa

2 whole ripe mangoes, peeled and diced
juice of 2 limes
½ cup orange juice
1 large red bell pepper, diced
½ tsp. five spice powder
½ Tbsp. minced shallots
¼ cup honey
1 tsp. creole seasoning

Mix together all ingredients. Refrigerate at least 1 hour to blend flavors.
Makes 8 servings, ¼ cup each.

Per Serving: 77 Calories

Protein 0 gr.	Carb. 20 gr.
Fat 0 gr.	Cal. from fat 0%
Chol. 0 mg.	Sodium 135 mg.

The Shellfish Myth

You may have heard that eating shellfish raises your cholesterol. Forget that thought: It's just a well-traveled rumor!

Shellfish can actually protect arteries and blood vessels by lowering bad-type blood cholesterol and providing the heart with many other protective functions. Shellfish is actually a heart champion. Up-to-date analysis shows low levels of cholesterol in oysters, mussels, clams and scallops. Crab and shrimp have slightly higher levels, though still modest amounts, and all are extremely low in fat.

The heart-healthy key is to cook and serve seafood without any added saturated fat such as butter or typical frying oils.

Pan-Seared Swordfish

swordfish (protein)
potatoes (complex carb.)
vegetables, salad (simple carb.)

Pan-Seared Swordfish With Mixed Vegetables

4 swordfish steaks (5 oz. each)
1 eggplant, sliced in ¼-inch slices
½ cup Lea and Perrins Worcestershire for Chicken
8 red-skinned potatoes, quartered
1 cup green beans, cut in 1-inch diagonal pieces, blanched
1 cup wax beans, cut in 1-inch diagonal pieces, thawed
1 tsp. olive oil
1 yellow bell pepper, cut into strips
1 red bell pepper, cut into strips
1 cup frozen sugar snap peas, thawed
1 tsp. creole seasoning
1 cup Herbal Vinaigrette (pg. 51)

Marinate swordfish and eggplant slices in Worcestershire sauce for up to 1 hour.

In a microwaveable dish, place potatoes, green beans and wax beans with ¼ cup water. Cover dish with plastic wrap and vent. Microwave on high for 4 to 5 minutes.

Spray large sauté pan with cooking spray; add oil and heat. Sauté marinated swordfish and eggplant on both sides until done. Remove fish. In same pan, sauté peppers for one minute. Add snap peas, then beans and potatoes, seasoning and Herbal Vinaigrette.

Serve the fish on top of the vegetables. Serves 4.

Per Serving: 345 Calories

Protein 28 gr.	Carb. 39 gr.
Fat 8.5 gr.	Cal. from fat 22%
Chol. 43 mg.	Sodium 502 mg.

Asian Daikon Salad

¼ cup rice wine vinegar
1 Tbsp. sesame oil
1 Tbsp. low-sodium soy sauce
¼ cup chicken stock (fat-free/low salt)
2 tsp. grated ginger root
½ tsp. creole seasoning
3 cups diagonally sliced daikon radishes (about 4 medium)
1½ cups sliced mushrooms (about 4 ounces)
⅓ cup sliced green onions
8 red leaf lettuce leaves
2 Tbsp. sesame seeds, toasted

In a tightly covered container, shake together vinegar, oil, soy sauce, stock, ginger root and seasoning. Pour over daikon slices, mushrooms and onions; toss until evenly coated. Cover and refrigerate until chilled, about 2 hours. Serve on lettuce leaves. Sprinkle with sesame seeds.

Makes 8 servings.

Per Serving: 47 Calories

Protein 1 gr.	Carb. 4 gr.
Fat 3 gr.	Cal. from fat 57%
Chol. 0 mg.	Sodium 152 mg.

Pan-Roasted Crab Cakes

crab (protein)
bread crumbs (complex carb.)
Tropical Salsa, salad (simple carb.)

Pan-Roasted Crab Cakes

1 lb. lump crabmeat*
3 Tbsp. light mayonnaise
2 cloves garlic, minced
½ cup egg substitute (or 2 eggs), lightly beaten
1 red bell pepper, diced fine
1 green bell pepper, diced fine
1 carrot, diced fine
1 tsp. creole seasoning
1 cup fine bread crumbs

* may substitute canned salmon, drained

● Serve with Tropical Salsa (pg. 55), ⅓ cup per serving.

Mix crabmeat with mayonnaise, garlic, egg substitute, vegetables, seasoning and bread crumbs. Shape into 8 cakes.

Spray a nonstick skillet with cooking spray; heat. Brown the cakes until golden brown and cooked through.

Place 2 warm crab cakes atop ⅓ cup of salsa on large plate. Serve Mixed Greens surrounding crab cake.

Serves 4.

Per Serving: 343 Calories

Protein 22 gr.   Carb. 48 gr.
Fat 7 gr.   Cal. from fat 18%
Chol. 15 mg.   Sodium 657 mg.

Mixed Greens With Citrus Vinaigrette

12 cups washed, dried and torn mixed greens (red leaf, romaine, frizee, radicchio, arugula or bibb)
½ cup Citrus Vinaigrette (pg. 52)
4 green onions, leaves curled
2 Tbsp. chopped fresh herbs (cilantro, basil, rosemary, thyme)
2 plum tomatoes, diced

Just before serving, toss lettuce leaves with Citrus Vinaigrette. Top with curly-leaved onion and sprinkle lightly with herbs and diced tomatoes.

Serves 4.

Per Serving: 71 Calories

Protein 3 gr.   Carb. 10 gr.
Fat 2 gr.   Cal. from fat 25%
Chol. 0 mg.   Sodium 79 mg.

Planning to Cook With Crabmeat?

Canned crab is available flaked or as lump or claw meat. Once opened, refrigerate and use within 2 days.

If canned crabmeat tastes metallic, let it soak in ice water for 5 minutes, then drain and blot before using.

Always use your fingers to pick through crabmeat—fresh or canned—to make sure no tiny pieces of shell were left in it.

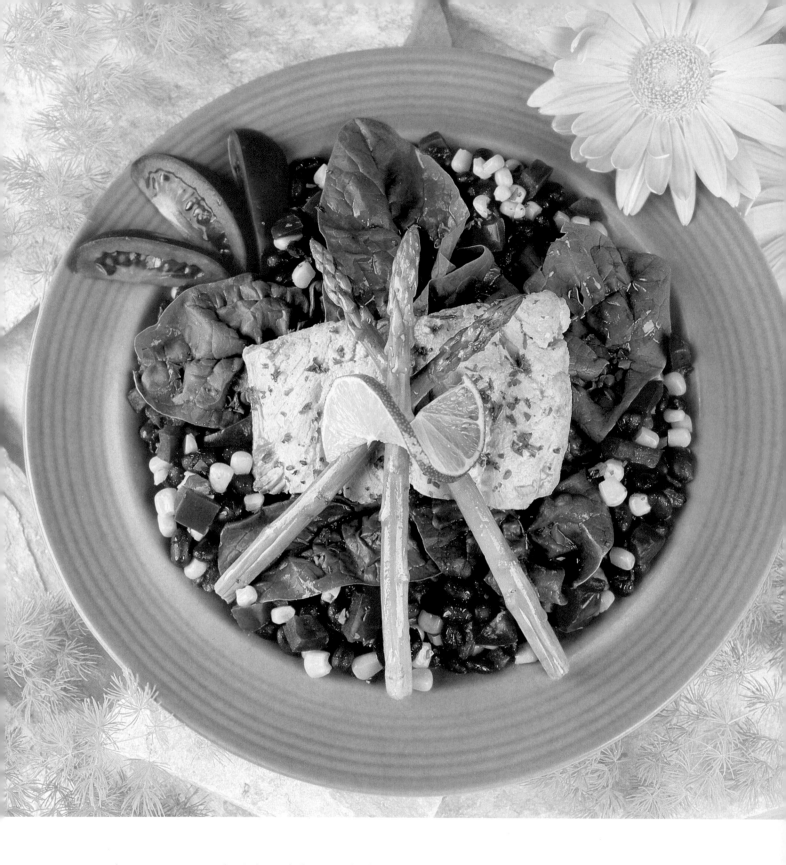

Salmon atop a colorful and flavorful Black Bean and Corn Salsa is tonight's main course, enhanced by the vivid colors and textures of spinach and asparagus—an unexpected yet delicious way to enjoy the subtle flavors of these vegetables. It's served with a Waldorf Salad in disguise—made over in a delightful way.

Poached Salmon

salmon, black beans (protein)
corn, black beans (complex carb.)
vegetables, fruit (simple carb.)

Poached Salmon Over Black Beans and Corn

Poaching stock:
- 1 cup white wine*
- 2 cups chicken stock (fat-free/low salt)
- 1 whole shallot, quartered
- 2 cloves garlic, minced
- 2 sprigs fresh thyme
- 2 bay leaves
- ¼ tsp. cracked black pepper
- ½ tsp. creole seasoning
- 4 salmon fillets (5 oz. each)
- 1 lb. asparagus, trimmed of tough stalks
- 2 cups Black Bean and Corn Salsa (pg. 55)
- 2 cups fresh spinach leaves, washed and stemmed
- 1 Tbsp. chopped chives
- 1 lemon, sliced

* or substitute dealcoholized wine or more chicken stock

In a large nonstick skillet, bring poaching stock to boil. Add salmon and asparagus spears; simmer 5 to 7 minutes until done.

Spoon Black Bean and Corn Salsa onto plate. Add fresh spinach leaves and place poached salmon and asparagus spears on top of the leaves.

Sprinkle with chopped chives and garnish with twisted lemon slice.

Serves 4.

Per Serving: 340 Calories

Protein 38 gr.	Carb. 38 gr.
Fat 4 gr.	Cal. from fat 11%
Chol. 51 mg.	Sodium 405 mg.

Waldorf Salad

- 2 large apples, cut into chunks
- ½ cup unsweetened pineapple chunks
- ½ stalk celery, chopped
- ½ cup carrots, shredded
- 1 small orange, peeled and sectioned
- ¼ cup golden raisins
- ¼ cup orange juice
- 1¼ cups nonfat vanilla yogurt
- 3 Tbsp. chopped walnuts

Combine all fruits along with vegetables and orange juice. Add yogurt, mixing well. Chill. Top with chopped walnuts for serving.

Makes 6 servings.

Per Serving: 114 Calories

Protein 2 gr.	Carb. 22 gr.
Fat 2 gr.	Cal. from fat 18%
Chol. 0 mg.	Sodium 53 mg.

Try Poaching

Poaching cooks food in simmering liquid. It produces a particularly delicate flavor in foods and keeps them moist.

Don't throw out a poaching liquid. It can be used either to make a sauce for the poached food or as a soup base.

If you're not going to use a poaching liquid within a couple of days, freeze it for up to six months. Be sure to label it though, so you don't have a mystery package!

Spicy Scallops and Cucumber Salad

scallops (protein)
roll (complex carb.)
vegetables (simple carb.)

Go Gourmet With Great-Tasting Garlic:

- One fresh medium garlic clove yields ½ tsp. minced garlic or ⅛ tsp. garlic powder or dried minced garlic.

- Crushing, mincing, pressing or purée-ing garlic releases essential oils and produces a more assertive flavor than slicing garlic cloves or leaving them whole.

- To give just a hint of flavor to a salad, rub a cut garlic clove in the bowl.

- Peel a garlic clove by placing the flat side of a large knife on top of a clove and giving it a gentle smack with your fist. The jolt will separate the skin from the clove for easy removal.

Spicy Scallops and Cucumber Salad

16 sea scallops, washed and drained
½ cup Lea and Perrins Worcestershire for Chicken
1 tsp. creole seasoning
2 tsp. Mrs. Dash seasoning
1 medium European cucumber, peeled, seeded and sliced diagonally
2 large tomatoes, seeded and cut into strips
1 large red onion, cut into strips
1 cup Cucumber Dill Dressing
4 cups mixed radicchio, bibb and endive lettuces
1 lemon, cut into wedges
2 Tbsp. chopped cilantro

Serve with whole-grain rolls or bread.

Marinate scallops in Worcestershire sauce for up to 1 hour. Toss scallops in seasonings. Spray a nonstick pan with cooking spray. Sear scallops in pan until cooked through.

Toss cucumbers, tomatoes and red onion in Cucumber Dill Dressing. Place salad on bed of lettuces. Drizzle one wedge of lemon juice over salad.

Add hot scallops to top of salad. Garnish with lemon wedge and chopped cilantro. Serve immediately with a whole grain roll.

Serves 4.

Per Serving: 299 Calories

Protein 27 gr.	Carb. 32 gr.
Fat 6 gr.	Cal. from fat 21%
Chol. 42 mg.	Sodium 502 mg.

Cucumber Dill Dressing

6 oz. fat-free cream cheese, softened
1½ oz. farmer's cheese
1 cup skim milk
1 cup cucumbers, peeled, seeded and chopped
1½ Tbsp. Dijon mustard
2 cloves garlic, minced
¼ tsp. cracked black pepper
1 tsp. creole seasoning
1 Tbsp. olive oil
juice of 1 lemon
½ tsp. Tabasco sauce
2 Tbsp. chopped fresh dill

Blend cheeses together with skim milk. Add remaining ingredients, except dill, and blend until smooth. Stir in dill.

Makes 1½ quarts, 24 servings, 4 Tbsp. each.

Per Serving: 38 Calories

Protein 1.5 gr.	Carb. 1 gr.
Fat 3 gr.	Cal. from fat 71%
Chol. 3 mg.	Sodium 34 mg.

Herbed Shrimp Pasta Primavera

shrimp, beans (protein)
pasta (complex carb.)
vegetables, salad (simple carb.)

Herbed Shrimp Pasta Primavera

1½ lbs. shrimp, peeled and deveined
¼ cup Lea and Perrins Worcestershire
    for Chicken
8 oz. dry bowtie pasta
2 tsp. olive oil
2 cloves garlic, minced
2 shallots, minced
1 each yellow, green and red bell
    peppers, cut into strips
1 tomato, cut into strips
1 cup broccoli florets, blanched
1 cup garbanzo beans
2 cups chicken stock (fat-free/low salt)
1 cup white wine*
1 tsp. creole seasoning
1 tsp. Mrs. Dash seasoning
⅓ cup shredded, part-skim mozzarella
    cheese
4 Tbsp. grated Parmesan cheese, divided
1 cup skim milk
2 Tbsp. chopped fresh herbs (cilantro,
    basil, rosemary, thyme)

* or substitute dealcoholized wine or more
   chicken stock

Marinate shrimp in Worcestershire sauce for at least 15 minutes.

In a large saucepan, cook bowtie pasta in salted water. Drain.

Spray a nonstick pan with cooking spray. Add olive oil and heat over medium-high heat. Lightly sauté garlic and shallots; add marinated shrimp and sauté 1 minute. Add vegetables, garbanzo beans, chicken stock, white wine and seasonings. Let cook for another 1 to 2 minutes until liquid reduces slightly. Mix together mozzarella and 2 Tbsp. of the Parmesan cheese.

Add to pan with skim milk and cooked pasta; toss to heat.

Sprinkle all with the remaining 2 Tbsp. grated Parmesan and the fresh herbs.

Serves 4.

Per Serving: 382 Calories

Protein 33 gr.	Carb. 52 gr.
Fat 5 gr.	Cal. from fat 12%
Chol. 209 mg.	Sodium 775 mg.

Caesar Salad

12 cups romaine lettuce, torn
½ cup Caesar Salad Dressing (pg. 53)

Toss lettuce with dressing. Serve immediately. Serves 4.

Per Serving: 54 Calories

Protein 2 gr.	Carb. 6 gr.
Fat 2.5 gr.	Cal. from fat 42%
Chol. 2.5 mg.	Sodium 60 mg.

More About Garlic

- *Minced garlic, purchased in a jar from the supermarket's produce section, takes advantage of the splendor of garlic without the chop-chop. The flavor is not the same, but the convenience may make up for the difference!*

- *Garlic cooks in about 30 seconds.*

- *If sautéing with onions, add the garlic at the end to keep it from becoming overbrowned and bitter.*

- *When roasted, garlic turns golden and butter-soft, with a mild, slightly sweet and nutty flavor.*

Tropical Seafood and Spinach Salad

seafood (protein)
bread (complex carb.)
spinach, peppers (simple carb.)

Even More About Garlic

- *Roast a whole head or individual cloves by trimming off stem ends and placing cut side down on pan sprayed with cooking spray. Loosely wrap in aluminum foil, drizzling with a scant teaspoon of olive oil and bake a 400 degrees for 25–30 minutes or until soft.*

- *Roast a half-dozen heads at one time; cool and squeeze out the individual cloves. Place the cloves in a freezer bag, press the bag flat and freeze. To use, pry off cloves with the tip of a knife; thaw for 1–2 minutes, mash and use.*

Tropical Seafood and Spinach Salad

8 oz. fresh white fish (snapper, grouper, sea bass or halibut), cut into chunks
1 lb. large shrimp
½ cup Jamaican Marinade (pg. 57)
2 red bell peppers, cut into chunks
12 oz. fresh spinach, washed and stemmed
3 oranges, peeled and sectioned
1 whole carrot, cut lengthwise into strips
1 cup Honey-Orange Vinaigrette (pg. 51)
2 tomatoes, diced fine
¼ cup dry-roasted pistachios, shelled

Marinate seafood in Jamaican Marinade for at least 1 hour. Put on wood skewers (which have been soaked in water) with red pepper chunks. Grill, basting with more marinade.

Toss spinach, oranges and carrot strips with Honey-Orange Vinaigrette. Spoon onto large plate; top with seafood skewer. Sprinkle with diced tomato and pistachios.

Serves 4.

Per Serving: 272 Calories

Protein 33 gr.	Carb. 26 gr.
Fat 4 gr.	Cal. from fat 13%
Chol. 186 mg.	Sodium 490 mg.

Focaccia Bread

2½ to 3 cups all-purpose flour
¾ cup chopped onions
1 Tbsp. olive oil
3 tsp. crushed dried rosemary leaves, divided
½ tsp. salt
½ tsp. cracked black pepper
1 pkg. of quick-acting dry yeast
2 cups very warm water (120 degrees)
2 to 2½ cups whole-wheat flour
Stone-ground cornmeal
1 tsp. olive oil

Mix 2 cups flour with onions, oil, 1 tsp. rosemary, salt, pepper and yeast in a large bowl. Add warm water. Use an electric mixer to beat on low for 1 minute, then medium for 1 minute, scraping the bowl frequently. Stir in remaining all-purpose flour, then whole-wheat flour, 1 cup at a time.

Turn dough onto lightly floured surface; gently roll in flour to coat. Knead about 10 minutes or until smooth and elastic. Spray large bowl with cooking spray. Place dough in bowl, turning to coat top. Cover and let rise in a warm place about 1 ½ hours or until double.

Spray jelly roll pan with cooking spray; sprinkle lightly with cornmeal. Punch down dough. Press into pan. Cover and let rise in warm place 30 minutes or until almost double.

Heat oven to 400 degrees. Press dough to edges of pan. Brush lightly with oil; sprinkle with 2 tsp. rosemary. Bake 30 to 35 minutes or until golden brown. Remove from pan. Cool on wire rack.

Makes 16 servings.

Per Serving: 135 Calories

Protein 4 gr.	Carb. 28 gr.
Fat 1 gr.	Cal. from fat 6%
Chol. 0 mg.	Sodium 70 mg.

Seafood and Pasta

seafood (protein)
pasta (complex carb.)
broccoli (simple carb.)

Mediterranean Seafood Stew

½ lb. large shrimp
6 oz. white fish (grouper, snapper or
  sea bass)
½ cup Lea and Perrins Worcestershire
  for Chicken
2 tsp. olive oil
2 cloves garlic, minced
1 small red onion, diced
2 cups chicken stock (fat-free/low salt)
4 cups Tomato Basil Sauce (pg. 59)
1 tsp. creole seasoning
2 Tbsp. chopped fresh herbs (cilantro,
  basil, rosemary, thyme)
juice of 1 lime
1 dozen clams, washed
1 dozen mussels, washed
10 oz. dry angel hair pasta
4 rosemary sprigs (optional)

Marinate shrimp and fish in Worcestershire sauce for up to 1 hour.

Spray large nonstick skillet with cooking spray. Add olive oil; heat. Add garlic and onion; sauté until translucent. Add shrimp and fish; lightly sauté. Add chicken stock, Tomato Basil Sauce, seasoning and fresh herbs; squeeze in juice of 1 lime. Add clams and mussels, and cook lightly until they open.

Meanwhile, cook angel hair pasta according to package directions. Drain. Serve 1 cup of pasta topped with an even portion of stew. Top with rosemary sprig.

Serves 4.

Per Serving: 418 Calories

Protein 42 gr.	Carb. 47 gr.
Fat 6 gr.	Cal. from fat 14%
Chol. 176 mg.	Sodium 555 mg.

Fresh Broccoli Salad

2 bunches fresh broccoli, trimmed and
  cut into small pieces
1 cup chopped fresh parsley
2 to 3 green onions, sliced
½ cup nonfat cottage cheese (or ricotta)
¼ cup light mayonnaise
½ cup skim milk
2 cloves garlic, minced
1 tsp. Mrs. Dash seasoning
½ tsp. creole seasoning
¾ tsp. dill weed

Blanch broccoli for 5 minutes in boiling water. Immerse quickly in ice water to chill; drain. Toss with parsley and green onions.

Make dressing by blending cottage cheese, mayonnaise, milk, garlic and seasonings in blender until smooth. Stir in dill. Toss with vegetables and chill well.

Makes 8 servings.

Per Serving: 76 Calories

Protein 3 gr.	Carb. 16 gr.
Fat 0 gr.	Cal. from fat 0%
Chol. 1 mg.	Sodium 54 mg.

Tips for Preparing Shrimp

Shell shrimp by holding the tail fin in one hand and peeling away the shell starting with the bottom "feet." The tail may be left on.

Generally, small to medium shrimp don't need deveining except for eye-appeal. However, the vein of larger shrimp will contain noticeable grit and should be removed.

Devein by cutting a shallow slit down the middle of the outside curve with a sharp, pointed knife. Pull out the dark vein, then rinse the slit under cold, running water.

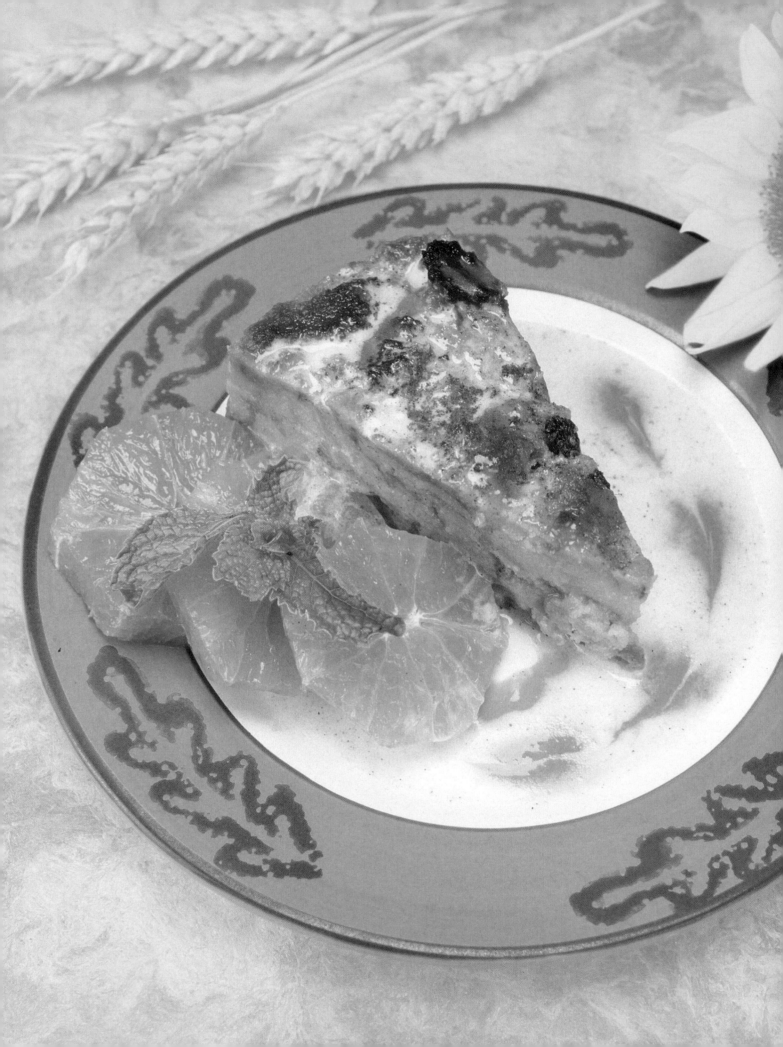

desserts
EIGHTEEN CHOICES

If you think healthy eating means a prison sentence, especially when it comes to desserts, these recipes will quickly change your mind. Nearly all of them have fewer than 150 calories per serving and are low in fat and cholesterol. They rely on the natural sweetness of fruits, using only small amounts of honey or sugar. What is left is the flavor—and lots of it!

Dessert is sometimes just a sweet afterthought, particularly if you've devoted all your culinary energy to the dishes that precede it. But creating something fresh and delicious doesn't have to be an ordeal.

There are lots of simple ideas that can jazz up your post-meal possibilities. Along with your time-tested favorite desserts, like bread pudding, you will also find many new and enticing ideas. Try them— you (and your guests) will love them!

Quick Refreshing Desserts

- Purée cubed peeled mango with a touch of lime juice in the food processor and chill. Serve atop pineapple chunks and strawberries.

- Scoop nonfat frozen yogurt onto a wedge of ripe cantaloupe or sliced mango.

Pictured: Pumpkin Bread Pudding (pg. 162)

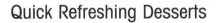

- Fold dried cherries, blueberries or cranberries into softened nonfat vanilla yogurt and refreeze.

- Top lemon sorbet with fresh raspberries and chunks of pineapple.

- Process 2 cans of undrained, unsweetened mixed fruit in a food processor until smooth. Freeze in a shallow pan, then return to processor until it's the consistency of sherbet.

- Pile fresh strawberries into large, stemmed balloon glasses, and add a generous splash of sparkling cider or champagne.

- Combine nonfat vanilla yogurt, all-fruit orange marmalade and a dash of cinnamon to make a dip for fresh peach slices.

On the following pages I offer eighteen more delicious dessert choices. From Chocolate Marble Cheesecake to Bavarian Cream, they prove that healthy desserts don't require sacrificing taste or pleasure.

desserts

Creamy Puddings

Pumpkin Bread Pudding

The Truth About Sugar

Health problems associated with sugar are controversial. The truth is this: Refined sugar has been shown to wreak havoc in the control of diabetes and hypoglycemia. It also raises triglycerides and the risk of dental cavities and obesity.

Sugar can cause a see-saw effect that can bring on the "more you have, the more you want" syndrome. It can lay the foundations for sugar dependency and abuse, and it sets a craving process in motion.

2 cups skim milk
1 cup honey
1 can (16 oz.) unsweetened pumpkin
½ tsp. ground ginger
1½ tsp. cinnamon
2 egg whites, slightly beaten
2 tsp. vanilla
⅓ cup dates, soaked in water and coarsely chopped
1 large carrot, grated
½ loaf French bread, cubed
2 Tbsp. fat-free frozen yogurt, thawed, per serving
sliced fruit for garnish
1 tsp. pourable fruit (purchased), per serving

Preheat oven to 350 degrees.
Mix together milk, honey, pumpkin, spices, egg whites, vanilla, dates and grated carrot.
Place bread cubes in a 9- x 13-inch pan sprayed with cooking spray. Pour liquid mixture over bread cubes.
Cover pan with foil and bake for 35 minutes. Remove foil and bake an additional 10 minutes or until browned on top. Cut into 15 squares. To serve place a square on a plate or in a sundae glass. Spoon on 2 Tbsp. yogurt as sauce. Garnish with fruit and drizzle with 1 tsp. all-fruit syrup.
Serves 15.

Per Serving: 154 Calories

Protein 3.5 gr.	Carb. 34 gr.
Fat 0 gr.	Cal. from fat 0%
Chol. 0 mg.	Sodium 130 mg.

Banana Pudding Soufflé

¾ cup polenta or coarse ground cornmeal
2 cups skim milk
1 cup puréed bananas
⅔ cup egg whites
2 Tbsp. sugar
cornmeal (to dust mold)
⅓ cup fat-free frozen yogurt

Whisk polenta into skim milk and cook according to package directions. Refrigerate overnight.
Preheat oven to 400 degrees.
Mix polenta with banana purée. Whip egg whites with sugar to a medium peak meringue. Gently fold into polenta mixture.
Spray five individual soufflé molds with cooking spray. Lightly dust with cornmeal. Divide mixture into the five molds. Place molds in a 9- x 13-inch pan filled with water. Bake until soufflés rise but are still creamy in center (about 30 minutes).
Top each with 1 Tbsp. fat-free frozen yogurt and serve immediately.
Serves 5.

Per Serving: 108 Calories

Protein 5 gr.	Carb. 22 gr.
Fat 0 gr.	Cal. from fat 0 %
Chol. 0 mg.	Sodium 56 mg.

Creamy Puddings (continued)

Rice Pudding

2 cups instant brown rice
¼ cup sugar
½ tsp. cornstarch
⅛ tsp. salt
3¼ cups skim milk
¼ cup raisins, dark or golden
1 tsp. cinnamon
2 tsp. vanilla
sprinkle of nutmeg

In a medium-sized saucepan, mix together rice, sugar, cornstarch and salt. Gradually stir in milk and bring to a simmer over medium-high heat, stirring constantly. Reduce heat to low and simmer slightly, stirring often, until rice is tender and pudding is creamy, about 5 minutes. Remove from heat and stir in raisins, cinnamon and vanilla.

Cover and let stand for 5 minutes or until ready to serve.

Spoon into individual bowls and sprinkle with nutmeg. May serve with fresh sliced peaches or other fruit.

Serves 6.

Per Serving: 166 Calories

Protein 6 gr.	Carb. 34 gr.
Fat 0 gr.	Cal. from fat 0%
Chol. 2 mg.	Sodium 116 mg.

Bavarian Cream

¾ cup pure maple syrup
1 cup skim-milk ricotta cheese
1½ cups nonfat plain yogurt
1 tsp. vanilla
2 tsp. unflavored gelatin
4 tsp. water

Mix maple syrup, ricotta cheese, yogurt and vanilla in blender. Whip until smooth, then empty into a large bowl.

Gently stir gelatin into water. Heat water slowly to dissolve gelatin.

Stir 1 Tbsp. of cheese and yogurt mixture into the warmed gelatin mixture. Stir in the remaining cheese and yogurt mixture until smooth. Chill overnight. Serve as a wonderful topping for fruit and other desserts.

Makes 15 servings, ¼ cup each.

Per Serving: 76 Calories

Protein 3 gr.	Carb. 12 gr.
Fat 0 gr.	Cal. from fat 0%
Chol. 6 mg.	Sodium 62 mg.

Make a Phyllo Tower

A beautiful way to serve Bavarian Cream or frozen sorbet is in a pastry tower.

To make, wrap a strip of aluminum foil around an 8-oz. can of tomato juice. Spray foil lightly with cooking spray. Cut phyllo sheets into 2½-inch widths and wrap sheets around foil, spraying each piece with more cooking spray. Take foil and dough off can and place on baking sheet. Repeat process to make 4 foil towers. Bake at 375 degrees for about 10 minutes or until browned. Let cool and remove foil.

Berry Banana Sundae

Cinnamon Tortilla Chips

2 burrito-sized, fat-free flour tortillas
2 tsp. cinnamon

Preheat oven to 400 degrees.
Cut tortillas into thin strips. Sprinkle the tortillas with cinnamon. Bake until crisp and lightly browned, about 3 minutes.
Makes 20 long strips; 2 strips per serving

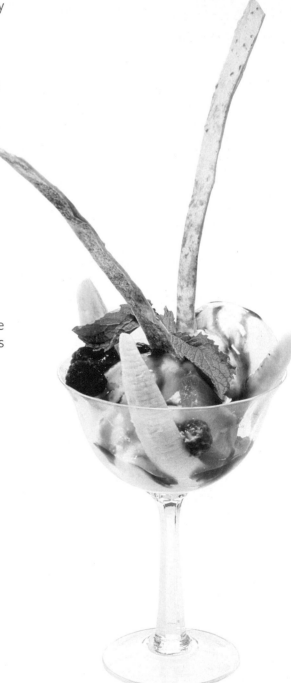

Natural Serving Bowls

Freshly fruited desserts are a sweet treat anytime of the year. To serve them with flair, use the serving bowls nature provides:

- *¹/₂ pineapple (sliced lengthwise, keeping the leaves intact)*

- *¹/₂ cantaloupe (scoop out the seeds and some melon)*

- *A large navel orange (slice off the top and scoop out the pulp)*

- *Bibb, green or red leaf lettuce leaves (serve as bed for fruit)*

Berry Banana Sundae

3 oz. scoop (¹/₃ cup) fat-free frozen
   vanilla yogurt
3 oz. scoop (¹/₃ cup) orange sorbet
2 Tbsp. raspberry pourable fruit
   (purchased)
4 fresh berries
3 orange sections
¹/₂ banana, cut lengthwise and into
   quarters
2 Cinnamon Tortilla Chips

Put yogurt and sorbet scoops into sundae glass. Top with sauce and fruit. Stand bananas on end against sides of glass.
Garnish with fruit and tortilla chips.
Serves 1.

Per Serving: 153 Calories

Protein 3 gr.   Carb. 35 gr.
Fat 0 gr.   Cal. from fat 0%
Chol. 0 mg.   Sodium 60 mg.

Fruit Finales

Warm Pears in Raspberry Sauce

½ cup seedless raspberry all-fruit
   spread
1 cup apple juice
2 tsp. grated lemon peel
2 Tbsp. lemon juice
3 firm bosc pears, peeled and cut into
   quarters

Mix all ingredients except pears in a 10-inch skillet. Add pears. Heat to boiling; reduce heat to medium-low. Simmer, uncovered, 30 minutes, spooning juice mixture over pears, and turning every 10 minutes until pears are tender.
   Serve warm or chilled.
   Makes 6 servings.

Per Serving: 84 Calories

Protein 0 gr.	Carb. 21 gr.
Fat 0 gr.	Cal. from fat 0%
Chol. 0 mg.	Sodium 16 mg.

Basket of Fresh Fruit

4 Wonton Cups
1 cup mixed fresh berries
4 oz. (or ½ cup) blueberries
2 kiwifruit, peeled and sliced
2 peaches, sliced
1 cup Strawberry Sauce (pg. 63)
¼ cup peach pourable fruit (purchased)

Place baked Wonton Cup on its side on plate and fill with one-fourth of the mixed berries. Arrange one-fourth of the other fruits around plate. Drizzle with one-fourth of the remaining strawberry sauce. Dot side of plate with one-fourth of the peach syrup. Repeat for remaining Wonton Cups and fruit.
   Serves 4.

Per Serving: 141 Calories

Protein 1 gr.	Carb. 35 gr.
Fat 0 gr.	Cal. from fat 0 %
Chol. 0 mg.	Sodium 34 mg.

Wonton Cups

6 wonton skins (purchased)

Spray a muffin pan with cooking spray. Place a wonton skin inside each muffin well, making sure all sides are covered.
   Bake on very low heat (225 degrees) for 4–6 minutes until lightly browned.
   Serves 6.

Per Serving: 24 Calories

Protein 1 gr.	Carb. 5 gr.
Fat 0 gr.	Cal. from fat 0 %
Chol. 0 mg.	Sodium 26 mg.

desserts
EIGHTEEN CHOICES

Presenting Perfect Pears

Bosc pears are perfect for poaching since they hold up well to heat. Firm Anjou pears can also be used. Remember—the sweeter and riper the pear, the sweeter the dessert.

Help pears ripen by placing them in a brown paper bag with a banana. The banana releases a gas that naturally sweetens the fruit. Pears are ripe when slightly soft around stem end. Refrigerate and use them within 3 to 5 days.

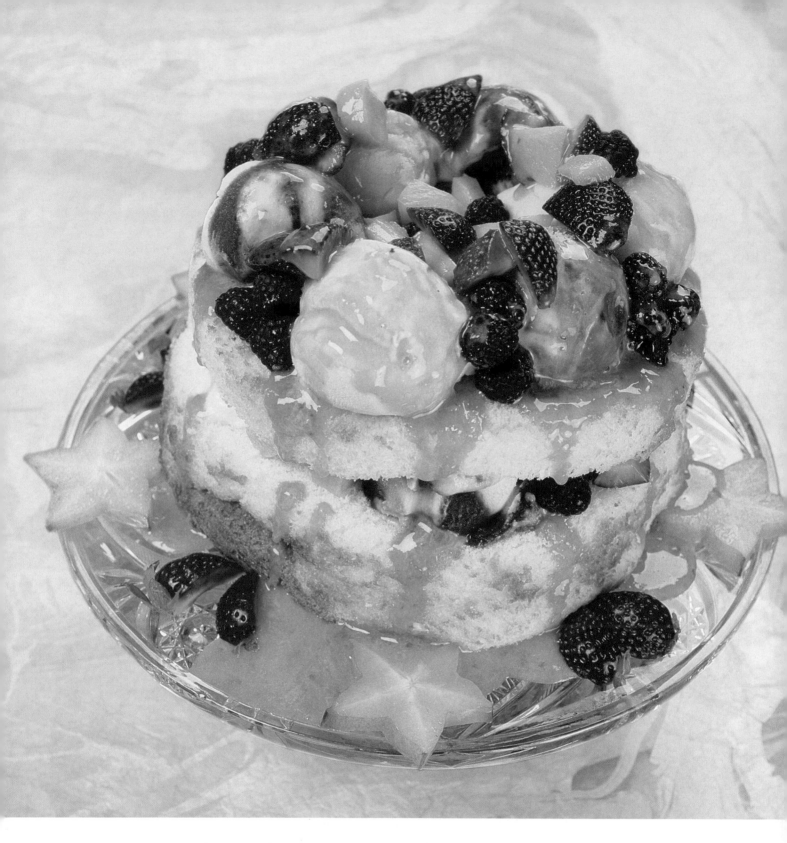

Sometimes dessert takes on a higher calling, the focus of the event itself. This festive offering of angel food cake filled and topped with tropical fruits and sorbets will bring oohs and aahs, as well as delight, whether it's topped with birthday candles or is simply a stand-up finish to a very special meal.

Cakes for Celebrations

Angel Food Celebration Cake

1 10-inch Angel Food Cake*
½ pt. frozen mango sorbet
½ pt. frozen raspberry sorbet
½ pt. fat-free frozen vanilla yogurt
1 mango, peeled and sliced
1 cup raspberries
2 cups strawberries, halved
¼ cup Strawberry Sauce (pg. 63)

* *You may use your favorite recipe or buy a prepared mix and follow package directions.*

Cut cake horizontally to make 2 layers. (To split, mark side of cake with toothpicks and cut with long, thin serrated knife.)

Immediately before serving, top bottom layer with alternating scoops of half the sorbets and frozen yogurt. (Work quickly—it melts!) Sprinkle with half of the sliced fruits. Place top layer of cake firmly on the bottom layer, then top with rounded scoops of remaining frozen products and sprinkle with remaining fruit.

Drizzle sauce over all.

Makes 12 servings.

Per Serving: 143 Calories

Protein 2 gr.	Carb. 25 gr.
Fat 1 gr.	Cal. from fat 1%
Chol. 0 mg.	Sodium 190 mg.

Brandied Pound Cake

½ cup strained apricot baby food (or ½ cup dried apricots, puréed with a little apple juice as needed until smooth)
½ cup canola oil
1 cup sugar
1½ cups egg substitute (or 6 eggs)
8 oz. fat-free cream cheese, softened
½ cup apricot brandy or nectar
1 tsp. rum extract
2 tsp. vanilla
1 tsp. orange extract
1 Tbsp. freshly squeezed lemon juice
2 cups cake flour
1 cup whole-wheat pastry flour
1 tsp. baking soda
1 tsp. baking powder
½ tsp. salt

Preheat oven to 325 degrees.

In a large mixing bowl, beat together apricot baby food and canola oil. Gradually add sugar, beating until creamy. Slowly add egg substitute while continuing to beat. Add softened cream cheese, brandy, extracts and lemon juice. Stir well.

In a separate bowl, combine flours, baking soda, baking powder and salt. Add the cream cheese mixture. Stir by hand until just blended. Pour batter into a 10-inch tube pan sprayed with cooking spray. Bake 1 hour and 20 minutes or until a toothpick inserted in the center comes out clean. Cool.

Serves 20.

Per Serving: 161 Calories

Protein 4 gr.	Carb. 25 gr.
Fat 5 gr.	Cal. from fat 27%
Chol. 0 mg.	Sodium 130 mg.

Healthy Modifications for Yummy Cakes

In a traditional cake, oil and eggs are the major players that interact with baking powder and baking soda to provide the cake's texture.

These are the changes I make that allow healthy modifications without compromising the flavor or texture: I replace whole eggs with liquid egg substitute or egg whites; I cut the amount of fat in half and change it to a monounsaturated oil; and I replace the missing half of the fat with a fruit purée like bananas, apricots, prunes and apples. I double the spices and flavorings since there is less fat to distribute the flavors.

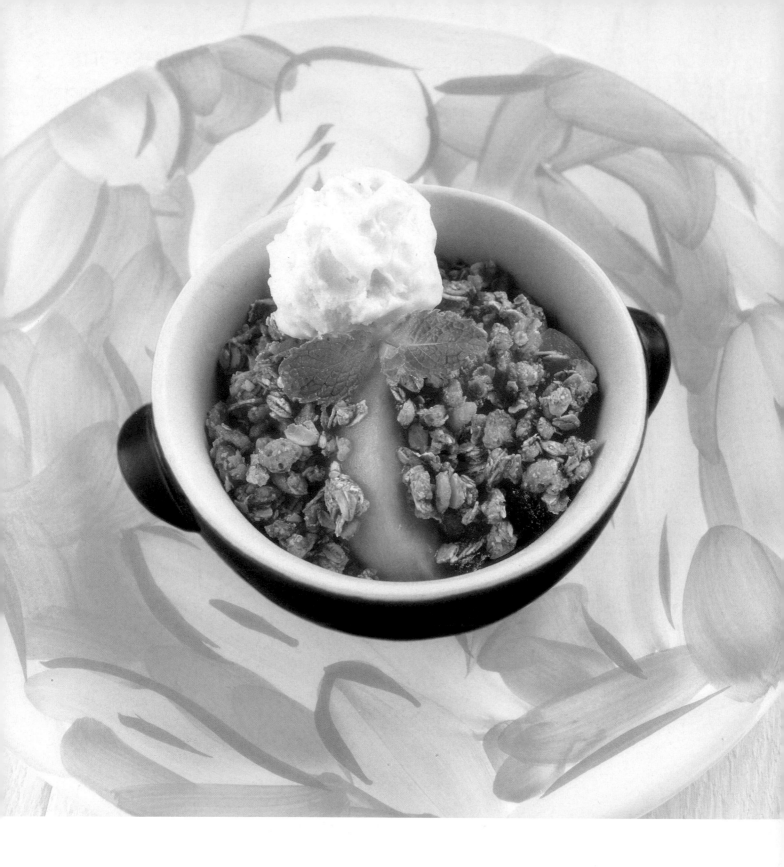

Luscious peaches topped with a nutty, crunchy topping and vanilla bean yogurt speak to us of summer, yet warm us in the winter. It's a scrumptious end to any meal.

Peach Delights

Peach Crisp

10 medium peaches, sliced (or 4 cans,
   15½ oz. each, unsweetened
   sliced peaches)*
¾ cup golden raisins
3 Tbsp. canola oil
3 Tbsp. honey
1 cup old-fashioned oats, uncooked
½ tsp. allspice
1 tsp. cinnamon
¼ tsp. salt
⅓ cup whole-wheat pastry flour
2 Tbsp. walnuts
½ cup unsweetened white grape juice

*   may substitute sliced apples. Then bake
    for 40 to 45 minutes.

Preheat oven to 375 degrees.

Spread half of peaches in a large rectangular pan; top with raisins. Heat together the oil and honey. Add oats, allspice, cinnamon, salt, flour and walnuts. Crumble half of this mixture onto the peaches in the pan. Cover with remaining peaches and the rest of topping. Pour grape juice over the top.

Bake uncovered for 25 minutes.

Makes 12 servings.

Per Serving: 158 Calories

Protein 2.5 gr.	Carb. 28 gr.
Fat 4 gr.	Cal. from fat 23%
Chol. 0 mg.	Sodium 46 mg.

Gingered Peach Melba

½ cup all-fruit raspberry spread
2 Tbsp. orange juice
½ tsp. ground ginger
4 ripe peaches, cut in half and pitted
   (or canned, unsweetened)
4 gingersnaps, crushed

Preheat oven to 425 degrees.

In a small microwaveable bowl, whisk together all-fruit spread, orange juice and ginger. Microwave for 2 to 3 minutes until thinned.

Place the peaches, cut side up, in a shallow 1-quart baking dish. Pour the gingered jam over the peaches and sprinkle with gingersnap crumbs. Bake for 15 to 20 minutes or until the peaches are tender when pierced with a knife and the syrup has thickened. Serve warm or at room temperature, with the sauce spooned over.

Serves 4.

Per Serving: 123 Calories

Protein 1 gr.	Carb. 27 gr.
Fat 1 gr.	Cal. from fat 7%
Chol. 0 mg.	Sodium 54 mg.

Sugar Substitutions

If a recipe doesn't rely on sugar for texture (like certain cakes and cookies), I have tried to eliminate or replace sugar with concentrated fruit juices, applesauce, puréed bananas, prunes or apricots.

I also sometimes replace sugar with honey or maple syrup. These are not perfectly healthy substitutions— they are still forms of sugar. The benefit is that they have a higher sweetness concentration so a smaller quantity may be used. For example, ¼ cup honey or maple syrup or ½ cup dried fruit purée will give the sweetness of 1 cup sugar; the addition of cinnamon or vanilla will enhance the sweetness of the dessert even more.

desserts

Pleasing Pies

Learning to Enjoy Less Sugar

Withdraw from sweets long enough to allow your blood sugar levels to stabilize and your energy and proper appetite for good foods to return. Choose fruit and desserts that are sweetened without sugar to satisfy your natural desire for a sweet taste.

Learning to enjoy foods with a lighter touch of sweetness and letting your taste buds change will transform your eating habits. Taste buds do change, but it takes time (about eight weeks). It's not easy, but it's worth it!

Beware of the tidal wave of sugar-free, fat-free desserts on the market. Usually the sugar has only been replaced with chemicals. These sweet treats will keep your taste buds from changing and leave you craving and desiring the "real thing."

Strawberry Yogurt Pie

1 can (20 oz.) unsweetened, crushed pineapple
1 envelope unflavored gelatin
1 cup fresh strawberries
1 1/2 cups nonfat plain yogurt
3 Tbsp. honey
2 tsp. lemon juice
1 tsp. vanilla
1 cup ripe mashed bananas

Drain pineapple, reserving juice. Set fruit aside. If needed, add unsweetened apple or white grape juice to reserved juice to make 3/4 cup. Pour into saucepan. Add gelatin and heat, stirring to allow gelatin to dissolve. Remove from heat and chill until partially set (like the consistency of unbeaten egg whites). Whip partially set gelatin with electric mixture till fluffy.

Set aside 1/3 cup pineapple and 3 whole strawberries.

Slice remaining strawberries. Mix together yogurt, honey, lemon juice and vanilla. Fold in remaining pineapple, sliced strawberries and mashed banana. Fold into whipped gelatin mixture and pour into cooled Healthy Graham Crust. Chill until firm.

Cut remaining strawberries and use with reserved pineapple as garnish just before serving.

Makes 8 servings.

Per Serving: 165 Calories

Protein 4 gr.	Carb. 36 gr.
Fat 1.5 gr.	Cal. from fat 8%
Chol. 3 mg.	Sodium 102 mg.

Healthy Graham Crust

2 Tbsp. reduced-calorie light butter
2 Tbsp. apricot all-fruit spread
3/4 cup fine graham cracker crumbs
1/3 cup Grape-Nuts cereal
1 tsp. cinnamon
1 Tbsp. brown sugar

Preheat oven to 375 degrees.

Spray a 9-inch pie plate with cooking spray. Set aside.

In a small saucepan, heat the butter and fruit spread just until melted.

In a medium bowl, stir together the cracker crumbs, cereal, cinnamon and sugar. Drizzle in the butter-fruit mixture. Using a fork, stir until well mixed.

Transfer the crumb mixture to the prepared pie plate. Using the back of a large spoon, press the crumb mixture firmly in the bottom and up the sides of the pie plate. Bake for 5 to 7 minutes or until the edges are lightly browned. Cool on a wire rack before filling.

Makes 1 pie crust; 8 servings.

Per Serving: 101 Calories

Protein 1 gr.	Carb. 20 gr.
Fat 2 gr.	Cal. from fat 18%
Chol. 2 mg.	Sodium 52 mg.

Pleasing Pies (continued)

Raisin Pie

1 box (15½ oz.) raisins
2¼ cups water
2 Tbsp. cornstarch
2 tsp. grated orange rind
¼ tsp. salt
2 Tbsp. orange juice
3 Tbsp. finely chopped walnuts
Phyllo Pastry Shell

Preheat oven to 350 degrees.
Boil raisins in 2 cups water for 5 minutes. Mix cornstarch into remaining ¼ cup cold water and add to raisins. Boil 1 minute more until thickened. Add remaining ingredients and pour into prepared pastry shell. Bake for 30 minutes.
Makes 10 servings.

Per Serving: 137 Calories

Protein 0 gr.	Carb. 32 gr.
Fat 1 gr.	Cal. from fat 6%
Chol. 0 mg.	Sodium 58 mg.

Phyllo Pastry Shell

1 package frozen phyllo dough

Preheat oven to 375 degrees.
Cut three sheets of phyllo dough in half to make 6 squares. Drape 1 square across a 9-inch pie plate. Press the phyllo into the plate and fold the overhanging edge toward the center, crumpling it slightly to fit. Lightly spray the dough with cooking spray. Repeat layering and spraying with the remaining squares. Bake for 4 to 6 minutes or until golden brown.
Makes 1 pastry shell, 8 servings.

Per Serving: 8 Calories

Protein 0 gr.	Carb. 2 gr.
Fat 0 gr.	Cal. from fat 0%
Chol. 0 mg.	Sodium 26 mg.

Pumpkin Pie

Brown sugar topping:
   ¼ cup packed brown sugar
   ¼ cup quick-cooking oats
   1 Tbsp. reduced-calorie light butter
1 can (16 oz.) pumpkin
1 can (12 oz.) evaporated skim milk
3 egg whites (or ½ cup egg substitute)
⅓ cup sugar
½ cup all-purpose flour
1½ tsp. pumpkin pie spice
¾ tsp. baking powder
⅛ tsp. salt
2 tsp. grated orange peel

Preheat oven to 350 degrees.
Prepare brown sugar topping by mixing the brown sugar, oats and butter together in a bowl. Set aside.
Spray 10-inch pie plate with cooking spray. Place remaining ingredients in blender or food processor in order listed. Cover and blend until smooth. Pour into pie plate. Sprinkle with topping.
Bake 50 to 55 minutes or until knife inserted in center comes out clean. Cool 15 minutes. Refrigerate about 4 hours or until chilled.
Makes 8 servings.

Per Serving: 157 Calories

Protein 6 gr.	Carb. 32 gr.
Fat less than 1 gr.	Cal. from fat 3%
Chol. 3 mg.	Sodium 144 mg.

Fun With Phyllo

Phyllo (also known as filo) is tissue-thin pastry dough. It's found in boxes in the frozen foods section at most supermarkets. Once opened, use phyllo within a few days.

Phyllo can be kept frozen for up to one year. Thaw frozen dough overnight in the refrigerator, and do not refreeze—it will become dry and brittle. It will also become dry and brittle if you don't work quickly, so don't remove it from its wrapping until you're ready to go. And keep those sheets you're not working on covered with wax paper topped by a damp cloth—it will keep it much more manageable. Just don't get the phyllo damp—it will become a soggy mess.

Pleasing Pies (continued)

Spiced Apple Cobbler Pie

2 tsp. fresh lemon juice
2 cups coarsely chopped apples
3 Tbsp. frozen apple juice concentrate, thawed
½ tsp. cinnamon
1 tsp. apple pie spice
1 cup whole-wheat pastry flour
½ cup sugar
2 tsp. baking powder
4 egg whites, lightly beaten
1 tsp. vanilla
½ cup chopped walnuts

Preheat oven to 325 degrees.

Lightly spray a square baking pan with cooking spray; set aside. Sprinkle the lemon juice over the apples, then add frozen juice concentrate, cinnamon and apple pie spice and toss gently until coated. Set aside.

In a large bowl, stir together the flour, sugar and baking powder. Then stir in the egg whites and vanilla. Add the apple mixture and walnuts (the mixture will be thick).

Transfer the mixture to the prepared baking pan. Bake about 35 minutes or until golden brown.

Makes 8 servings.

Per Serving: 149 Calories

Protein 4 gr.	Carb. 28 gr.
Fat 2.5 gr.	Cal. from fat 15%
Chol. 0 mg.	Sodium 113 mg.

Summertime Fruit Pizza

1 burrito-sized fat-free flour tortilla
cinnamon
4 oz. fat-free cream cheese
¼ cup honey
1 tsp. vanilla
¼ cup fat-free ricotta cheese
3 kiwi, peeled and sliced
1 cup strawberries, sliced
1 peach or nectarine, sliced
¼ cup all-fruit apricot spread, warmed

Preheat oven to 375 degrees.

Spray a pizza pan with cooking spray. Place tortilla on pan; sprinkle lightly with cinnamon. Bake about 4 to 5 minutes until edges begin to lightly brown. Remove from oven and cool.

Beat together the cream cheese, honey and vanilla, then beat in the ricotta cheese till smooth. Spread the cheese mixture atop the cooled crust. Arrange the kiwi, strawberries and peaches on top, slightly overlapping. Chill in the refrigerator while preparing glaze.

Microwave the apricot spread in a small microwaveable bowl on high for 1 minute. Using a clean pastry brush, brush the glaze over the fruit. Chill 1 hour before serving.

Makes 6 servings.

Per Serving: 124 Calories

Protein 3 gr.	Carb. 28 gr.
Fat less than 1 gr.	Cal. from fat 3%
Chol. 0 mg.	Sodium 53 mg.

Delicious Cheesecake

Chocolate Marble Cheesecake

1 cup Yogurt Cheese (see right column)
1 ½ cups reduced-fat chocolate graham cracker crumbs
3 Tbsp. apricot all-fruit spread, melted
1 cup skim-milk ricotta cheese
4 egg whites
1 pkg. (8 oz.) light cream cheese
1 Tbsp. unbleached flour
1 tsp. vanilla
½ cup sugar
¼ cup unsweetened Dutch-process cocoa
1 tsp. almond extract

Preheat oven to 350 degrees.

Prepare Yogurt Cheese; set aside. Coat a 9-inch springform pan with cooking spray. In a bowl, mix graham cracker crumbs and all-fruit spread. Lightly press crumb mixture into bottom of pan. Bake for 8 minutes. Set aside. Increase oven temperature to 375 degrees.

Process ricotta cheese in a food processor until almost smooth. Add egg whites and process until smooth. Add Yogurt Cheese, cream cheese, flour, vanilla and half of sugar. Process until a smooth batter forms. Pour half of filling into a bowl. Add cocoa, remaining sugar and almond extract. Stir until well combined.

Alternately pour batters, half of each at a time, into crust. Gently swirl batters with a spatula.

Bake until a knife inserted in center comes out clean, 35 to 40 minutes. Cool on wire rack for 15 minutes. Run a knife blade around the edge of pan. Cool for 30 minutes. Remove side from pan. Cool completely. Chill for at least 4 hours.

Cut into 12 slices.

Per Serving: 100 Calories

Protein 6 gr.	Carb. 17 gr.
Fat 1 gr.	Cal. from fat 9%
Chol. 1 mg.	Sodium 69 mg.

Orange-Blueberry Cheesecake

3 cups Yogurt Cheese (see right column)
5 gingersnaps, crushed
2 packages (8 oz. each) fat-free cream cheese
½ cup sugar
¼ cup egg substitute (or 2 eggs)
4 egg whites
2 Tbsp. frozen orange juice concentrate, thawed
1 Tbsp. grated orange rind
1 tsp. orange extract
½ cup blueberry all-fruit spread

Preheat oven to 350 degrees.

Prepare Yogurt Cheese; set aside. Spray a 10-inch springform pan with cooking spray. Sprinkle crushed gingersnaps evenly over bottom of pan.

Blend cream cheese and sugar in food processor until light and fluffy. Add Yogurt Cheese and process until smooth. Add egg substitute, egg whites, orange juice concentrate, orange rind and orange extract. Process until mixture is well blended.

Spoon mixture over crushed gingersnaps. Bake for 35 minutes (center will be soft but firm when chilled). Remove from oven, and let cool to room temperature on a wire rack. Cover and chill 4 hours or until set.

Spread blueberry all-fruit spread evenly over top of cheesecake. Cover and chill 1 hour.

Makes 14 servings.

Per Serving: 117 Calories

Protein 8 gr.	Carb. 19 gr.
Fat 0 gr.	Cal. from fat 0%
Chol. 2 mg.	Sodium 93 mg.

Try Making Yogurt Cheese

Low-fat yogurt cheese is easy to make and has a rich, creamy consistency that's just right for making cheesecakes, dips and spreads. To make yogurt cheese, simply line a strainer with cheesecloth and spoon in nonfat plain yogurt (with active cultures). Place the strainer over a deep bowl and refrigerate for 24 hours. Two cups of yogurt make 1 ½ cups of cheese.

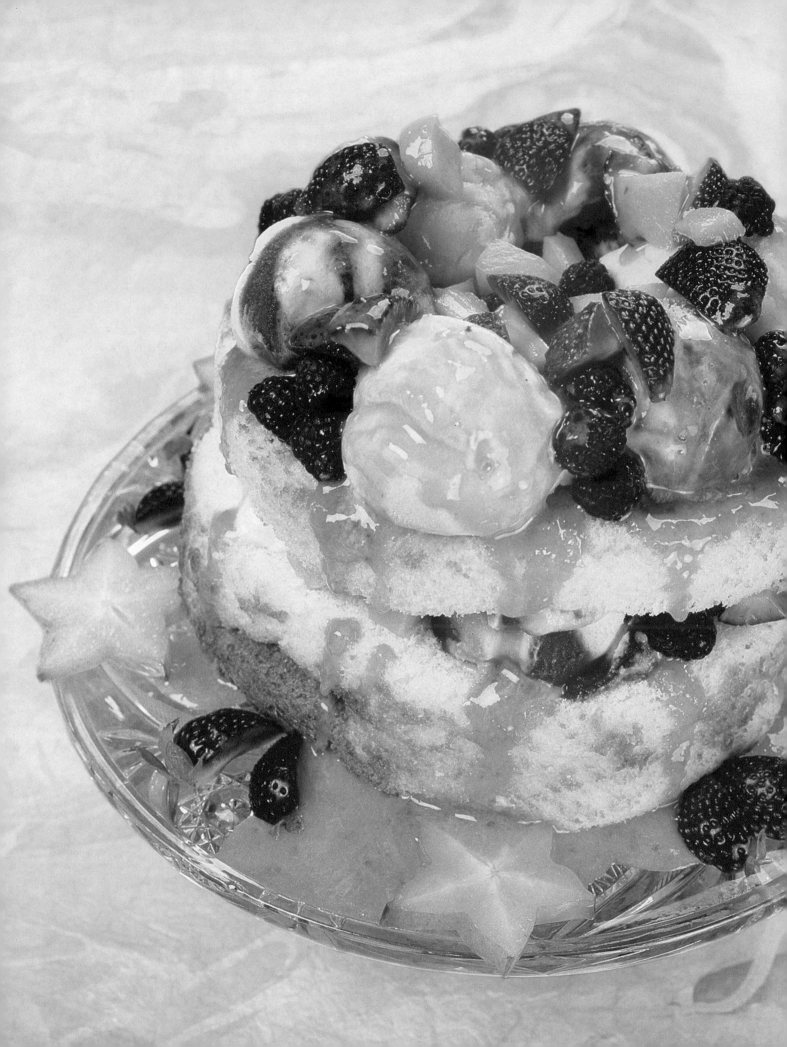

entertain with style

There's nothing like the holidays to bring out the worst in our old eating habits and attitudes about food. For centuries holidays have centered around the sharing of food. The good news is that a lifestyle of good health doesn't mean eliminating food from your holiday celebrations. Learn how to prepare old, unhealthy classics in new healthy ways. Add some guaranteed-to-please new favorites.

Throwing a Great Party

Effortless entertaining allows you to enjoy your party, delight in your guests and savor delicious food. Here are some basic tips to keep it simple, and keep it fun. My best friend calls it "partying without Prozac."

- Develop a nonfussy menu with one main item, for example: a pork tenderloin, or Red Lentil Chili, plus several salads.

- When people ask you what to bring, tell them *exactly what you want*, for example: a fresh vegetable platter, fresh grapes or berries, sparkling water or whole-grain breads or rolls.

- Designate a helper to restock food items, change CDs, check on candles and help with party pacing.

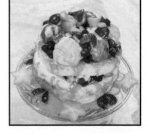

- A buffet is the easiest and most popular way to serve at a party, especially for a small space. Arrange the table with stacks of plates at the beginning of the buffet. Place your silverware, napkins and beverages at the end—or have them already placed at the dinner table—to allow your guests to keep their hands free to serve themselves.

- Think about traffic flow. Spread food around the house so people don't congregate in one room. (It's always the kitchen in my house!) Have several food areas, including a beverage, appetizer or dessert station, in another area of the house or adjacent to the table.

- Set the mood with candles, lighting and music.

- Plan a cleanup after the party, such as watching a funny video with the few friends or family that stay to help clean up.

Pictured: Angel Food Celebration Cake (page 193)

A Traditional Holiday Dinner

Antipasto Cups With Creamy Herb Dip
Roast Turkey With Gravy
Turkey Gravy
Cranberry Chutney

Cornbread Dressing
Sweet Potato Casserole
Green Beans and Mushrooms
Mom's Tropical Fruit Salad

Antipasto Cups With Creamy Herb Dip

2 medium red bell peppers
2 medium yellow bell peppers
2 medium green bell peppers
2 medium carrots, quartered and cut into 3-inch strips (or shaved baby carrots)
1 medium zucchini, quartered and cut into 3-inch strips
12 radish roses (pg. 30, garnishing tips)
12 scallion brushes (pg. 30, garnishing tips)
6 pepperoncini peppers
2 oz. part-skim mozzarella, cubed
1 ½ cups Creamy Herb Dip (pg. 61)

Cut the top off each pepper, reserving it for other uses; remove seeds. Cut a thin slice from the bottom of each pepper, if necessary, to help the pepper stand upright to become a cup for the remaining ingredients.

Arrange equal amounts of cut carrots, zucchini, radishes, onion fans, peppers and cheese in each pepper cup. Chill thoroughly. Serve with Creamy Herb Dip.

Serves 6.

Per Serving: 90 Calories

Protein 8 gr.	Carb. 10 gr.
Fat 2 gr.	Cal. from fat 20%
Chol. 6 mg.	Sodium 205 mg.

Roast Turkey With Gravy

1 whole turkey, thawed
celery leaves
thin onion slices
garlic cloves

Before roasting, place a thin layer of celery leaves and thin slices of onion between the skin and the breast meat of the turkey. This will add rich flavor to the meat and absorb much of the fat from the skin.

Roast turkey according to package directions, basting with lower-salt chicken stock.

One serving is 3 oz. turkey.

Per Serving: 158 Calories

Protein 27 gr.	Carb. 0 gr.
Fat 5.5 gr.	Cal. from fat 34%
Chol. 72 mg.	Sodium 180 mg.

A Traditional Holiday Dinner (continued)

Turkey Gravy

turkey giblets
1 qt. water
1 onion, cut in pieces
1 stalk celery, cut in pieces
2 Tbsp. canola oil
2 cloves garlic, minced
1 Tbsp. cornstarch
1 bay leaf
$1/2$ cup white wine*
1 tsp. Mrs. Dash seasoning
$1/2$ tsp. salt
$1/4$ tsp. cracked black pepper

* or substitute dealcoholized wine or chicken stock

First, make turkey stock. Remove the giblets from the bird and wash well. Boil giblets together with neck in 1 quart of water with onion and celery. Drain off broth and refrigerate to defat.

To make gravy, heat canola oil in a medium saucepan. Add garlic and cook for 30 seconds. Stir in cornstarch until smooth. Add 3 cups turkey stock, bay leaf, wine and seasonings. (Purchased or homemade chicken stock may be substituted for turkey stock.) Cook over low heat, stirring, until gravy thickens, about 5 minutes. Remove bay leaf.

Makes 15 servings, $1/4$ cup each.

Per Serving: 20 Calories

Protein 0 gr.	Carb. 0 gr.
Fat 2 gr.	Cal. from fat 100%
Chol. 0 mg.	Sodium 120 mg.

Cranberry Chutney

2 cups chopped fresh cranberries
1 cup peeled, chopped Granny Smith apples
3 Tbsp. brown sugar
2 Tbsp. chopped prunes
2 Tbsp. chopped onions
$1/2$ tsp. ground cinnamon
$1/4$ tsp. five spice powder
$1/3$ cup apple-cranberry juice
3 Tbsp. red wine vinegar
2 tsp. lemon juice

Combine all ingredients in a medium saucepan. Bring mixture to a boil. Cover, reduce heat and simmer for 30 minutes, stirring frequently. Uncover and cook, stirring, for 5 minutes or until mixture is thickened.

Makes 8 servings, $1/3$ cup each.

Per Serving: 84 Calories

Protein 0 gr.	Carb. 21 gr.
Fat 0 gr.	Cal. from fat 0%
Chol. 0 mg.	Sodium 15 mg.

A Traditional Holiday Dinner (continued)

Cornbread Dressing

1 cup finely chopped celery
½ cup chopped onions
2 Tbsp. snipped fresh parsley
  (or 2 tsp. dried)
1 tsp. ground sage
1 ½ tsp. poultry seasoning
½ tsp. cracked black pepper
½ tsp. salt
2 packages (12 oz. each) unseasoned
  cornbread stuffing cubes
3 cups chicken stock (fat-free/low salt) or
  homemade turkey stock (pg. 177)
½ cup egg substitute (or 4 egg whites)

Preheat oven to 350 degrees.

Lightly spray a medium nonstick skillet with cooking spray. Add the celery and onions. Cook over medium heat until tender. Stir in herbs, seasoning and spices.

Lightly spray a large casserole dish with cooking spray. Place the cornbread cubes in casserole. Add onion and celery mixture, 2 cups of the broth and egg substitute. Gently toss. Drizzle with remaining broth to moisten bread thoroughly; gently toss again to mix well.

Bake uncovered for 30 to 40 minutes or until heated through.

Makes 10 servings.

Per Serving: 135 Calories

Protein 4 gr.	Carb. 27 gr.
Fat 1 gr.	Cal. from fat 6%
Chol. 0 mg.	Sodium 320 mg.

Sweet Potato Casserole

3 cups cooked and cubed sweet
  potatoes
¼ cup sugar
4 egg whites
1 tsp. vanilla
1 tsp. cinnamon
Topping:
  ½ cup brown sugar
  3 Tbsp. flour
  1 Tbsp. melted butter
  ¼ cup chopped pecans

Preheat oven to 350 degrees.

Spray a 1 ¼-quart casserole dish with cooking spray. Set aside until ready to use.

In a food processor or with electric mixer, mix potatoes, sugar, egg whites, vanilla and cinnamon. Spoon into prepared casserole dish.

Make topping by rubbing together, with your fingers, the brown sugar, flour and butter until crumbly. Stir in pecans. Sprinkle the mixture on top of sweet potatoes.

Bake approximately 30 minutes until golden brown.

Makes 8 servings.

Per Serving: 178 Calories

Protein 5 gr.	Carb. 31 gr.
Fat 3.5 gr.	Cal. from fat 18%
Chol. 1 mg.	Sodium 188 mg.

entertain with style

Green Beans and Mushrooms

2 lbs. green beans
2 tsp. olive oil
2 cloves garlic, minced
2 Tbsp. minced shallots
½ tsp. dried basil
½ tsp. dried rosemary
½ tsp. Mrs. Dash seasoning
2 Tbsp. chopped fresh parsley
½ tsp. creole seasoning
½ lb. (8 oz.) fresh mushrooms, trimmed
2 Tbsp. Lea and Perrins Worcestershire for Chicken

Trim ends from green beans; break into smaller pieces if desired. Steam in chicken stock until crisp tender.

Spray nonstick skillet with cooking spray; add olive oil and heat over medium-high heat. Add garlic and shallots; cook for about 1 minute. Add herbs and seasonings, and sauté another 30 seconds; then add mushrooms and Worcestershire sauce. Continue to sauté for about 3 to 4 minutes, then add steamed green beans. Toss together and serve.

Makes 8 servings.

Per Serving: 53 Calories

Protein 2 gr.   Carb. 9 gr.
Fat 2 gr.   Cal. from fat 17%
Chol. 0 mg.   Sodium 229 mg.

Mom's Tropical Fruit Salad

1 large can (28 oz.) unsweetened, crushed pineapple
2 packets of unflavored gelatin
4 cups unsweetened white grape juice
2 packages (8 oz. each) fat-free cream cheese
1 small can of mandarin oranges, rinsed and drained

Drain pineapple, reserving juice. Set fruit and juice aside.

In a medium saucepan, add gelatin to 1 cup white grape juice and let dissolve. Place pan on burner and gently heat on medium-high, adding remaining juice and drained juice from canned pineapple. Stir constantly, and remove from heat as the mixture begins to thicken. Add two packages of softened cream cheese and beat with electric mixer or in food processor. Add pineapple and mandarin oranges.

Let chill 3 to 4 hours or until firm. Cut into pieces to serve.

Makes 16 servings.

Per Serving: 68 Calories

Protein 4 gr.   Carb. 13 gr.
Fat 0 gr.   Cal. from fat 0%
Chol. 15 mg.   Sodium 125 mg.

More Lower Calorie Favorites

Calories and/or fat are reduced by using egg whites instead of whole eggs; by lowering the amount of sugar and adding cinnamon instead; by lowering the amount of butter and adding flour to thicken; by using fewer nuts; and by using cooking spray rather than butter.

The original fruit salad recipe contained 336 calories and 13 grams of fat (38 percent of calories). The new version, with no added sugar, is trimmed down to only 68 calories and 9 grams of fat (0 percent of calories).

Calories, sugar and/or fat are reduced by using unflavored gelatin and 100 per-cent pure juice instead of already flavored gelatin products, and by using fat-free cream instead of whipped topping and cottage cheese.

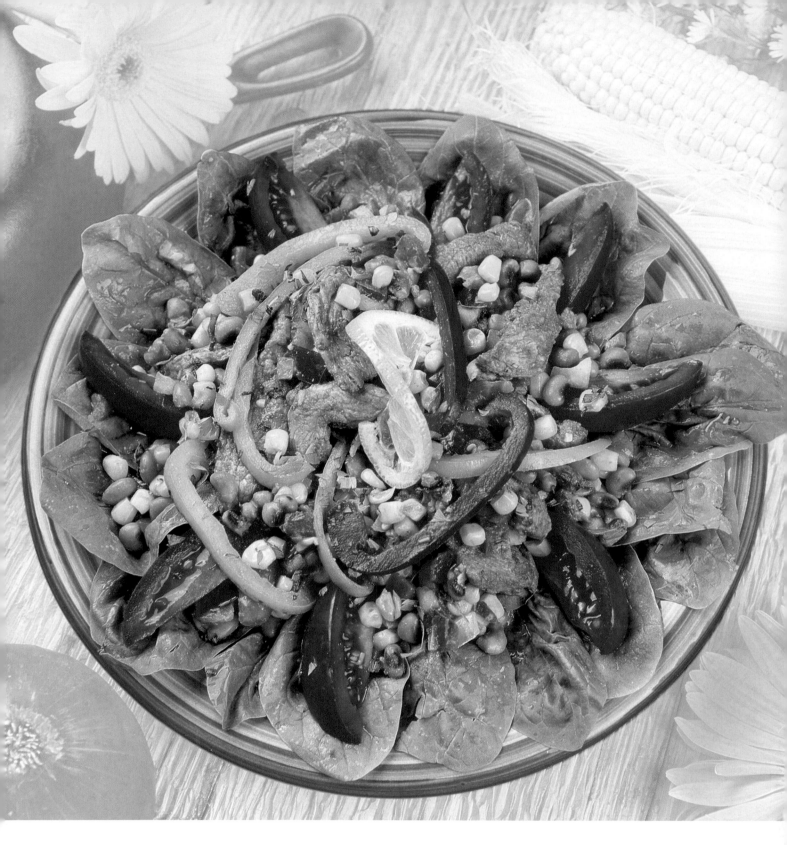

A dish of pork and black-eyed peas is soul food in the South—the original comfort food and a traditional New Year's menu item. Lean and tender pork is combined with the black-eyed peas and spinach, becoming a new version of a time-tested favorite.

New Year's Brunch

Bran Muffins With Date Cream Cheese Spread
Fiesta Cheese Cloud
Seared Pork and Black-Eyed Pea Salad
Orange-Blueberry Cheesecake

Bran Muffins With Date Cream Cheese Spread

skim milk or yogurt (protein)
muffin (complex carb.)
raisins (simple carb.)

¼ cup unprocessed wheat bran
¼ cup unprocessed oat bran
⅓ cup boiling water
½ cup milk
3 Tbsp. packed brown sugar
3 Tbsp. canola oil
3 Tbsp. honey
4 egg whites (or ½ cup egg substitute)
1⅓ cups whole-wheat pastry flour
2 tsp. baking powder
1 tsp. cinnamon
¼ tsp. salt
½ cup raisins

- Serve in large basket with cream cheese spread in bowl in center.

Preheat oven to 400 degrees.

Spray the bottoms in a 12-well muffin tin with cooking spray or line with paper baking cups.

Mix brans and boiling water; set aside. In medium bowl, beat milk, brown sugar, oil, honey and egg whites. Add bran mixture, flour, baking powder, cinnamon and salt; stir until moistened (batter will be lumpy). Fold in raisins.

Divide batter evenly among muffin cups. Cups will be about two-thirds full. Bake 20 to 25 minutes or until golden brown. Immediately remove from pan.

Makes 12 muffins.

Per Serving: 138 Calories

Protein 4 gr.	Carb. 24 gr.
Fat 3 gr.	Cal. from fat 23%
Chol. 0 mg.	Sodium 71 mg.

Date Cream Cheese Spread

2 pkgs. (8 oz. each) fat-free or
light cream cheese
8 oz. unsweetened pitted dates,
chopped
2 Tbsp. skim milk
½ cup walnuts, chopped

Process all ingredients in a food processor or blender until mixed evenly. Transfer to airtight container and store in refrigerator for up to 2 weeks.

Serving size: 3 Tbsp.

Per Serving: 64 Calories

Protein 4 gr.	Carb. 12 gr.
Fat 1 gr.	Cal. from fat 14%
Chol. 15 mg.	Sodium 151 mg.

New Year's Brunch (continued)

Fiesta Cheese Cloud

cheese, eggs, milk, bacon (protein)
bread (complex carb.)
strawberries (simple carb.)

12 slices whole-wheat bread
½ lb. turkey bacon, chopped
2 Tbsp. grated red onion
2 cloves garlic, minced
8 oz. grated part-skim mozzarella/
 part-skim cheddar cheese blend
1 cup egg substitute (or 4 eggs)
2½ cups skim milk
1 Tbsp. Dijon mustard
½ tsp. creole seasoning
1 tsp. Mrs. Dash seasoning
1 small can of green chilies, chopped

- Make several, based on crowd size—
  serve from the stove, right out of the
  oven.

Preheat oven to 325 degrees.

Trim crusts from bread cut in half into triangular shapes. Arrange 12 of the triangles in bottom of a 12- x 8-inch greased baking dish.

In a nonstick skillet, sauté bacon until crisp. Remove from pan and drain on paper towel. Add onion and garlic to pan, and sauté until transparent.

Sprinkle turkey bacon and half of grated cheese onto bread slices in pan, then top with sauté onion and garlic. Add remaining bread slices.

Beat eggs; add milk, mustard and seasonings; add chilies (with liquid). Pour liquid over casserole and let stand at room temperature for 1 hour (or even refrigerate overnight if more convenient). Bake 1 hour; serve immediately.

Serves 8.

Per Serving: 249 Calories

Protein 22 gr.	Carb. 23 gr.
Fat 7 gr.	Cal. from fat 17%
Chol. 39 mg.	Sodium 545 mg.

Seared Pork and Black-Eyed Pea Salad

1 lb. pork tenderloin or medallions,
 cut into strips
½ cup Balsamic Marinade (pg. 56)
2 cloves garlic, minced
1 each red and green bell peppers,
 quartered
2 cups Black-Eyed Pea and Corn Salad
12 oz. fresh spinach, washed and
 stemmed
1 Tbsp. chopped fresh herbs (cilantro,
 basil, rosemary, thyme)
2 plum tomatoes, quartered

- Black-eyed peas are the traditional
  good luck meal for New Year's—this
  dish gives a new twist to the classic!
  Serve on a large family style platter.

Marinate pork strips in ¼ cup Balsamic Marinade for up to 1 hour.

Spray a nonstick skillet with cooking spray. Add garlic and lightly sauté. Add pork to skillet, sautéing 2 to 3 minutes until no pink remains. Add the remaining marinade, the peppers and the Black-Eyed Pea and Corn Salad to skillet, lightly tossing to heat.

Line plate with spinach; top with pork salad mixture, allowing peppers to lie on top. Garnish with herbs and tomato quarters.

Serves 4.

Per Serving: 304 Calories

Protein 32 gr.	Carb. 31 gr.
Fat 7 gr.	Cal. from fat 21%
Chol. 78 mg.	Sodium 332 mg.

New Year's Brunch (continued)

Black-Eyed Pea and Corn Salad

16 oz. (or 2 cups frozen) black-eyed peas
¼ cup chicken stock (fat-free/low salt)
1 cup frozen corn kernels, thawed
2 plum tomatoes, diced
¾ red onion, minced
1 serrano pepper, minced
2 Tbsp. finely chopped cilantro
1 tsp. olive oil
4 cloves garlic, minced
juice of 1 lime
¼ cup Balsamic Marinade (pg. 56)
1 tsp. cumin
2 tsp. hot pepper sauce
1 tsp. creole seasoning

Follow package instructions to cook black-eyed peas in ¼ cup chicken stock; cool. Combine all ingredients. Allow to marinate at least one hour.

Makes 8 servings, ½ cup per serving.

Per Serving: 85 Calories

Protein 4 gr.	Carb. 15 gr.
Fat 1 gr.	Cal. from fat 10%
Chol. 0 mg.	Sodium 170 mg.

Orange-Blueberry Cheesecake

3 cups Yogurt Cheese (pg. 173)
5 gingersnaps, crushed
2 packages (8 oz. each) fat-free cream cheese
½ cup sugar
¼ cup egg substitute (or 2 eggs)
4 egg whites
2 Tbsp. frozen orange juice concentrate, thawed
1 Tbsp. grated orange rind
1 tsp. orange extract
½ cup blueberry all-fruit spread

- Simply delicious!

Preheat oven to 350 degrees.

Prepare Yogurt Cheese; set aside. Spray a 10-inch springform pan with cooking spray. Sprinkle crushed gingersnaps evenly over bottom of pan.

Blend cream cheese and sugar in food processor until light and fluffy. Add Yogurt Cheese and process until smooth. Add egg substitute, egg whites, orange juice concentrate, orange rind and orange extract. Process until mixture is well blended.

Spoon mixture over crushed gingersnaps. Bake for 35 minutes (center will be soft but firm when chilled). Remove from oven, and let cool to room temperature on a wire rack. Cover and chill 4 hours or until set.

Spread blueberry all-fruit spread evenly over top of cheesecake. Cover and chill 1 hour.

Makes 14 servings.

Per Serving: 117 Calories

Protein 8 gr.	Carb. 19 gr.
Fat 0 gr.	Cal. from fat 0%
Chol. 2 mg.	Sodium 93 mg.

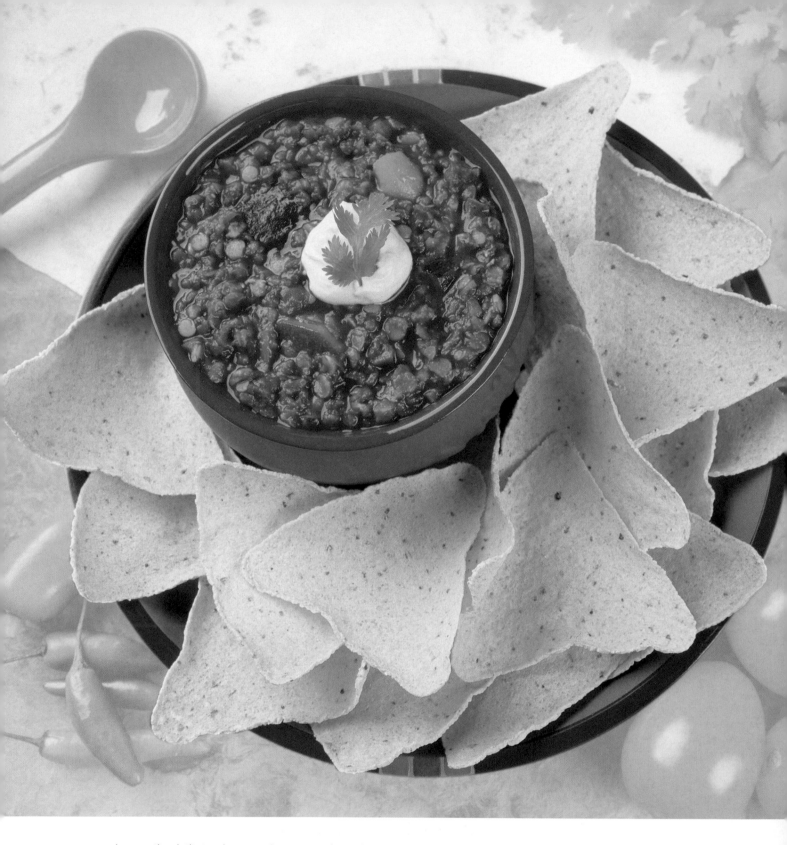

Red Lentil Chili is the perfect "¡Hola!" for your Super Bowl Mexican Buffet. Cook up a recipe of this delicious, mouth-watering chili and serve it in individual bowls with baked tortilla chips. Your crew will cheer for this dish—it has the winning score!

Super Bowl Mexican Buffet

Red Lentil Chili
Crunchy Jicama and Melon Salad
Chicken Quesadillas
Spicy Tomato Salsa

Black Bean and Corn Salsa
Turkey Tortilla Roll
Berry Banana Sundae With
Cinnamon Tortilla Chips

Red Lentil Chili

½ lb. carrots
1 small zucchini
1 small yellow squash
½ large eggplant
½ large red onion
¾ Tbsp. olive oil
12 oz. bag red or brown lentils, rinsed
2 cups chicken stock (fat-free/low salt)
1 tsp. Mrs. Dash seasoning
1 tsp. creole seasoning
2 bay leaves
½ Tbsp. oregano
½ tsp. cumin
1 tsp. chili powder
¾ tsp. cayenne
¾ tsp. nutmeg
2 cloves garlic, minced
1 jalapeño pepper, chopped
2 cans (32 oz. each) plum tomatoes

- Serve in fondue pot over flame with small mugs.

In food processor, finely chop carrots, zucchini, squash, eggplant and onion. Spray nonstick skillet with cooking spray. Add olive oil. Heat over medium high heat. Add chopped vegetables. Sauté for 5 minutes. Add lentils, chicken stock, seasonings, herbs, spices, garlic, jalapeño peppers and tomatoes. Simmer for 2 hours.
Makes 10 servings, 1 ½ cups each.

Per Serving: 134 Calories

Protein 8 gr.	Carb. 26 gr.
Fat 1 gr.	Cal. from fat 8%
Chol. 0 mg.	Sodium 406 mg.

Crunchy Jicama and Melon Salad

1 medium jicama, julienned
1 medium cantaloupe, cut into ½-inch cubes
3 Tbsp. lime juice
3 Tbsp. chopped fresh mint (or 1 Tbsp. dried)
1 tsp. grated lime peel
2 tsp. honey
¼ tsp. salt

- Serve in Mexican Pottery Bowl.

In a medium-sized bowl, mix together all ingredients. Cover and refrigerate 2 hours or until chilled.
Makes 4 servings.

Per Serving: 62 Calories

Protein 1 gr.	Carb. 15 gr.
Fat 0 gr.	Cal. from fat 0%
Chol. 0 mg.	Sodium 91 mg.

Super Bowl Mexican Buffet (continued)

Chicken Quesadillas

1 medium onion, sliced
½ large green bell pepper, diced
½ large red bell pepper, diced
2 Tbsp. chicken stock (fat-free/low salt)
1 tsp. minced garlic
8 large mushrooms, cleaned and sliced
⅛ tsp. cumin
⅛ tsp. crushed red pepper
pinch cayenne pepper
2 Tbsp. rice wine vinegar
1 tsp. chopped fresh cilantro
1 lb. boneless, skinless chicken breast
1 tsp. Mrs. Dash seasoning
1 tsp. creole seasoning
6 burrito-sized, fat-free flour tortillas
¾ cup grated part-skim cheddar
    cheese
1 cup mixed lettuces
2 cups Black Bean and Corn Salsa
3 Tbsp. nonfat sour cream
½ cup Spicy Tomato Salsa

- Grill several quesadillas, cut into wedges, place on platter and serve with salsa and nonfat sour cream in center of platter.

Spray a nonstick skillet with cooking spray and heat. Add onion, peppers and chicken stock and quickly sauté. Add garlic, mushrooms, cumin, chili powder and cayenne pepper. Cook for 2 minutes, stirring frequently. Add vinegar and cilantro, and cook until most of the liquid evaporates, about 2 minutes.

Sprinkle chicken breasts with seasonings and grill. Cut crosswise into ½-inch strips.

Lay each tortilla on surface of another hot nonstick skillet or griddle. Put 2 Tbsp. vegetable mixture, 2 oz. chicken (½ cup) and 2 Tbsp. cheese on one half of each tortilla. Fold over, and grill until browned and crispy and cheese is melted.

Cut each quesadilla into 3 triangles and lay on plate next to lettuce. Top lettuce with ⅓ cup Black Bean and Corn Salsa. Serve with ¼ cup salsa topped with ½ Tbsp. nonfat sour cream.

Makes 6 servings, 3 triangles per serving.

Per Serving: 431 Calories

Protein 42 gr.	Carb. 50 gr.
Fat 7 gr.	Cal. from fat 15%
Chol. 84 mg.	Sodium 599 mg.

Spicy Tomato Salsa

1½ lbs. plum tomatoes, seeded and
    diced
½ cup finely diced red onion
1 jalapeño, stemmed, seeded and finely
    diced
1 Tbsp. chopped fresh cilantro
1 tsp. cumin
1 tsp. creole seasoning
¼ tsp. cracked black pepper
2 cloves garlic, minced
juice of 1 lime

Combine all ingredients in a medium-sized bowl. Refrigerate to allow flavors to blend.

Use 2 Tbsp. per serving.

Per Serving: 15 Calories

Protein 0 gr.	Carb. 3 gr.
Fat 0 gr.	Cal. from fat 0%
Chol. 0 mg.	Sodium 160 mg.

Super Bowl Mexican Buffet (continued)

Black Bean and Corn Salsa

2 cups black beans, drained and rinsed
1 cup frozen corn kernels, thawed
2 plum tomatoes, diced
½ red onion, minced
1 serrano pepper, minced
1 Tbsp. chopped fresh cilantro
1 Tbsp. olive oil
4 cloves garlic, minced
juice of 2 limes
1 Tbsp. balsamic vinegar
1 tsp. cumin
2 tsp. hot pepper sauce
1 tsp. creole seasoning

- Serve in large bowl in center of platter, surrounded by chips.

In a large bowl, combine all ingredients and mix well. Allow to marinate at least one hour before serving.

Makes 10 servings, ⅓ cup each.

Per Serving: 79 Calories

Protein 4 gr.   Carb. 13 gr.
Fat 1.5 gr.   Cal. from fat 17%
Chol. 0 mg.   Sodium 118 mg.

Turkey Tortilla Roll

2 Tbsp. Black Bean Dip* (pg. 61)
2 Tbsp. fat-free sour cream
1 burrito-sized fat-free flour tortilla
1 cup shredded mixed lettuces
2 oz. turkey breast, sliced
4 strips red bell peppers
4 strips green bell peppers
2 tomato slices
⅓ cup Pineapple Tomato Salsa (pg. 55)

* *may use purchased dip or make Black Bean Dip*

- Make a number of rolls, rolled tightly, and cut into pinwheels; serve overlapped on platter.

Spread Black Bean Dip and fat-free sour cream onto tortilla to cover. Top with lettuce, turkey, peppers and tomatoes.

Roll tortilla tightly burrito style, secure with toothpicks and cut in half.

Serves 1.

Per Serving: 262 Calories

Protein 24 gr.   Carb. 37 gr.
Fat 2 gr.   Cal. from fat 7%
Chol. 40 mg.   Sodium 433 mg.

Super Bowl Mexican Buffet (continued)

Cinnamon Tortilla Chips

2 burrito-sized, fat-free flour tortillas
2 tsp. cinnamon

Preheat oven to 400 degrees.
Cut tortillas into thin strips. Sprinkle the tortillas with cinnamon. Bake until crisp and lightly browned, about 3 minutes.
Makes 20 long strips; 2 strips per serving

Berry Banana Sundae

3 oz. scoop (⅓ cup) fat-free frozen
   vanilla yogurt
3 oz. scoop (⅓ cup) orange sorbet
2 Tbsp. raspberry pourable fruit
   (purchased)
4 fresh berries
3 orange sections
½ banana, cut lengthwise and into
   quarters
2 Cinnamon Tortilla Chips

• Serve when your team wins—
  or doesn't!

Put yogurt and sorbet scoops into sundae glass. Top with sauce and fruit. Stand bananas on end against sides of glass.
Garnish with fruit and tortilla chips.
Serves 1.

Per Serving: 153 Calories

Protein 3 gr.   Carb. 35 gr.
Fat 0 gr.   Cal. from fat 0%
Chol. 0 mg.   Sodium 60 mg.

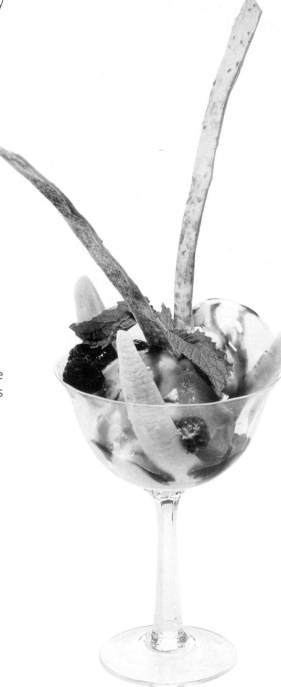

Valentine's Day Romantic Dinner

Balsamic Chopped Tomatoes
Salad of Mixed Greens
Cucumber Dill Dressing

Chicken Au Poivre
Strawberry Yogurt Pie

Balsamic Chopped Tomatoes

2 medium ripe tomatoes, chopped
1 medium red bell pepper, chopped
1 medium yellow bell pepper, chopped
1 small red onion, chopped
2 tsp. capers
3 Tbsp. chopped fresh basil
1 Tbsp. balsamic vinegar
2 tsp. freshly squeezed lemon juice
2 cloves garlic, minced
1 tsp. dried oregano
1/2 tsp. creole seasoning
freshly ground black pepper to taste
1 recipe of Garlic Toast (pg. 126)

Mix together all ingredients but garlic toast in a large bowl; cover and refrigerate 1 hour.
Equally divide and place on a mound of salad on each serving plate with 1 slice hot garlic toast alongside.
Serves 4.

Per Serving: 121 Calories

Protein 4 gr.   Carb. 24 gr.
Fat 1 gr.   Cal. from fat 11%
Chol. 0 mg.   Sodium 310 mg.

Salad of Mixed Greens

12 cups washed, dried and torn mixed
   greens (red leaf, romaine,
   frizee, radicchio, arugula or bibb)
1/2 cup Citrus Vinaigrette (pg. 52)
4 green onions, leaves curled
2 Tbsp. chopped fresh herbs (cilantro,
   basil, rosemary, thyme)
2 plum tomatoes, diced

• Serve with Cucumber Dill Dressing.

Just before serving, toss lettuce leaves with Citrus Vinaigrette. Top with curly-leaved onion and sprinkle lightly with herbs and diced tomatoes.
Serves 4.

Per Serving: 71 Calories

Protein 3 gr.   Carb. 10 gr.
Fat 2 gr.   Cal. from fat 25%
Chol. 0 mg.   Sodium 79 mg.

Cucumber Dill Dressing

6 oz. light cream cheese
1/3 cup farmer's cheese
1 cup skim milk
1 cup cucumbers, peeled, seeded and
   chopped
1 1/2 Tbsp. Dijon mustard
2 cloves garlic, minced
1/4 tsp. cracked black pepper
1 tsp. creole seasoning
1 Tbsp. olive oil
juice of 1 lemon
1/2 tsp. Tabasco
2 Tbsp. chopped fresh dill

Blend cheeses and skim milk in a blender. Add all other ingredients except the dill and blend until smooth. Stir in dill.
Makes 24 servings, 4 Tbsp. each.

Per Serving: 38 Calories

Protein 1.5 gr.   Carb. 1 gr.
Fat 3 gr.   Cal. from fat 71%
Chol. 3 mg.   Sodium 34 mg.

Valentine's Day Dinner (continued)

Chicken Au Poivre

Make this delicious basil sauce to serve with your favorite chicken recipes.

1/2 cup white wine*
2 Tbsp. chopped fresh basil
2 Tbsp. lemon juice
1/2 tsp. cracked black pepper

* or substitute dealcoholized wine or chicken stock (fat-free/low salt)

Mix together all ingredients. Makes 10 servings, 1 Tbsp. each.

4 boneless, skinless chicken breast halves (1 lb.)
1 tsp. cracked black pepper
1/2 tsp. Mrs. Dash seasoning
1 tsp. olive oil
2 cloves garlic, minced
1 small red onion, finely chopped
1/4 cup fennel, sliced into 1/2-inch slices
1/4 cup sun-dried tomatoes, slivered
2 tsp. capers, rinsed
2 cups cooked orzo
2 shiitake mushrooms, sliced
1 cup white wine*
2 cups chicken stock (fat-free/low salt)
2 Tbsp. lemon juice
4 leaves basil
1 tsp. creole seasoning

* or substitute dealcoholized wine or more chicken stock

- **Serve with Orzo and Basil Sauce**

Rub chicken with pepper and Mrs. Dash. Grill over hot coals, or sear in hot skillet until done. Set aside.

Spray nonstick skillet with cooking spray. Add olive oil and heat on medium high. Sauté garlic, onion and fennel until all begin to soften, about 3 to 4 minutes. Add sun-dried tomatoes, capers and orzo; stir. Add mushrooms, white wine, chicken stock, lemon juice, basil and creole seasoning. Cook gently for another 3 to 4 minutes or until liquids begin to reduce. Pour entire mixture, including juice, onto plate.

Top with the grilled chicken and 1 Tbsp. of Basil Sauce per serving.

Serves 4.

Per Serving: 340 Calories

Protein 32 gr.	Carb. 36 gr.
Fat 7.5 gr.	Cal. from fat 20%
Chol. 72 mg.	Sodium 820 mg.

Strawberry Yogurt Pie

1 can (20 oz.) unsweetened, crushed pineapple
1 envelope unflavored gelatin
1 1/2 cups nonfat plain yogurt
3 Tbsp. honey
2 tsp. lemon juice
1 tsp. vanilla
1 cup fresh strawberries
1 cup ripe mashed bananas

- **Make in heart-shaped cake pan rather than a pie plate.**

Drain pineapple, reserving juice. Set fruit aside. If needed, add unsweetened apple or white grape juice to reserved juice to make 3/4 cup. Pour into saucepan. Add gelatin and heat, stirring to allow gelatin to dissolve. Remove from heat and chill until partially set (like the consistency of unbeaten egg whites). Whip partially set gelatin with electric mixture till fluffy.

Set aside 1/3 cup pineapple and 3 whole strawberries.

Slice remaining strawberries. Mix together yogurt, honey, lemon juice and vanilla. Fold in remaining pineapple, sliced strawberries and mashed banana. Fold into whipped gelatin mixture and pour into cooled Healthy Graham Crust (pg. 170). Chill until firm.

Cut remaining strawberries and use with reserved pineapple as garnish just before serving.

Makes 8 servings.

Per Serving: 165 Calories

Protein 4 gr.	Carb. 36 gr.
Fat 1.5 gr.	Cal. from fat 8%
Chol. 3 mg.	Sodium 102 mg.

Easter Dinner

Eggplant Rollatini
Apple Walnut Salad
Cornish Game Hens

Risotto With Spring Vegetables
Cheesy Cornsticks
Angel Food Celebration Cake

Eggplant Rollatini

1 lb. fresh spinach, washed and
    stemmed
¾ lb. eggplant, peeled and cut
    lengthwise into thin slices
½ onion, finely chopped
2 cloves garlic, minced
¼ tsp. creole seasoning
1 tsp. Mrs. Dash garlic herb seasoning
2 Tbsp. chopped fresh Italian parsley
1 Tbsp. chopped fresh basil
16 oz. skim milk ricotta cheese
½ cup feta cheese, crumbled
1 Tbsp. grated Parmesan cheese
⅓ cup dry bread crumbs (purchased)
1 egg (or ¼ cup egg substitute)
1 egg white, slightly beaten
4 cups Tomato Basil Sauce (pg. 59)

- Serve one rollatini per person on
  pool of tomato basil sauce.

Preheat oven to 400 degrees.

Steam spinach until wilted. Drain well and roughly chop. Reserve. Spray each side of eggplant slices with cooking spray. Bake 10 minutes, flip over and finish baking until tender. Reserve. Reduce oven temperature to 350 degrees.

Spray nonstick skillet with cooking spray. Sauté onions and garlic, adding spinach at end. Let cool. Add seasonings, herbs, cheeses and bread crumbs. Mix in egg and egg white. Chill.

To make rollatini, place 2 heaping tablespoons of spinach-cheese mixture on each eggplant slice. Roll up and place open end down in casserole dish. Cover with 1 cup Tomato Basil Sauce. Bake for 30 minutes.

Place 3 rollatini on each plate. Top with ¾ cup heated Tomato Basil Sauce.

Serves 4.

Per Serving: 309 Calories

Protein 30 gr.	Carb. 23 gr.
Fat 5 gr.	Cal. from fat 15%
Chol. 21 mg.	Sodium 785 mg.

Apple Walnut Salad

2 Granny Smith apples, cored and
    sliced thin
2 Tbsp. chopped walnuts
2 Tbsp. chicken stock (fat-free/low salt)
1 Tbsp. white wine vinegar
2 tsp. walnut oil (or olive oil)
1 Tbsp. finely chopped shallots
1 tsp. Dijon mustard
¼ tsp. salt
¼ tsp. cracked black pepper
8 cups washed, dried and torn mixed
    greens (red leaf, romaine, frizee,
    radicchio, arugula or bibb)

In a small, dry skillet over low heat, stir walnuts until lightly toasted, about 3 minutes. Transfer to a plate to cool.

In a large salad bowl, whisk together chicken stock, vinegar, oil, shallots, mustard, salt and pepper. Add greens and apples and toss thoroughly. Sprinkle with the toasted walnuts.

Per Serving: 91 Calories

Protein 2.5 gr.	Carb. 14 gr.
Fat 4 gr.	Cal. from fat 35%
Chol. 0 mg.	Sodium 159 mg.

Easter Dinner (continued)

Cornish Game Hens on Risotto With Spring Vegetables

2 Cornish hens, halved lengthwise
2/3 cup Lea and Perrins Worcestershire for Chicken
2 cloves garlic, minced
2 Tbsp. chopped fresh rosemary
1 tsp. Mrs. Dash seasoning
1/2 tsp. creole seasoning

Preheat oven to 375 degrees.

Remove skin from Cornish hens where possible. Place in small roasting pan and top with remaining ingredients. Let marinate for at least 1 hour.

Place hens in oven for 45 minutes or until juices run clear when pierced with fork. Brush occasionally with Worcestershire sauce in pan. See picture for beautiful plate presentation.

Serves 4.

Per Serving: 150 Calories

Protein 25 gr.   Carb. 0 gr.
Fat 4 gr.   Cal. from fat 28%
Chol. 74 mg.   Sodium 202 mg.

Risotto With Spring Vegetables

5 1/2 to 6 1/2 cups chicken stock
   (fat-free/low salt)
16 baby carrots, shaved and cut in half
8 medium stalks asparagus, trimmed
   and cut into 2-inch pieces
1 cup sugar snap peas (thawed if frozen)
1 red bell pepper, cut into strips
2 tsp. olive oil
2 cloves garlic, minced
1 red onion, diced
1 cup arborio rice, uncooked

1/2 cup white wine*
1/2 tsp. creole seasoning
1 1/2 Tbsp. chopped fresh basil
1/2 cup grated Parmesan cheese
2 Tbsp. chopped fresh herbs (cilantro, basil, rosemary, thyme)

* or substitute dealcoholized wine or more chicken stock

In a medium-sized stockpot, bring chicken stock to boil over medium heat. Add carrots and cook 3 to 5 minutes until almost tender. Add asparagus and snap peas, and cook 1 minute longer. Remove vegetables with slotted spoon and place in bowl to cool. Reduce heat and keep stock simmering.

Spray a nonstick skillet with cooking spray. Add olive oil; heat. Add garlic and onions, and sauté until translucent, about 3 minutes. Add rice and stir to coat grains. Add wine and cook until most of liquid has been absorbed, about 2 to 3 minutes. Add 1/2 cup simmering chicken stock and cook another 2 to 3 minutes.

Continue adding stock, 1/2 cup at a time, until rice begins to soften, about 15 minutes.

Stir in the seasoning and basil, adding more stock to keep mixture creamy. Stir in reserved vegetables and cheese. Sprinkle with herbs.

Serves 4.

Per Serving: 316 Calories

Protein 13 gr.   Carb. 52 gr.
Fat 7 gr.   Cal. from fat 19%
Chol. 10 mg.   Sodium 393 mg.

Easter Dinner (continued)

Cheesy Cornsticks

⅓ cup skim milk
2 egg whites, lightly beaten
1 Tbsp. olive oil
⅓ cup whole-wheat pastry flour
½ cup stone-ground cornmeal
¼ cup grated Parmesan cheese
2 tsp. baking powder
½ tsp. sugar
¼ tsp. salt

Preheat oven to 425 degrees.

Spray a muffin pan or cast-iron cornstick mold with cooking spray.

Combine milk, egg whites and oil in a measuring cup; stir briskly with a fork until mixed. In a medium-sized bowl, whisk together flour, cornmeal, cheese, baking powder, sugar and salt. Make a well in the center of the dry mixture and pour in the milk mixture. Stir until just combined.

Spoon a heaping tablespoon of the batter into each of 8 cornstick molds or divide the batter among 4 muffin cups. Bake for 10 to 12 minutes or until set and lightly browned.

Makes 8 cornsticks.

Per Serving: 83 Calories

Protein 4 gr.	Carb. 10 gr.
Fat 3 gr.	Cal. from fat 32%
Chol. 2 mg.	Sodium 231 mg.

Angel Food Celebration Cake

1 10-inch Angel Food Cake*
½ pt. frozen mango sorbet
½ pt. frozen raspberry sorbet
½ pt. fat-free frozen vanilla yogurt
1 mango, peeled and sliced
1 cup raspberries
2 cups strawberries, halved
¼ cup Strawberry Sauce (pg. 63)

* *You may use your favorite recipe or buy a prepared mix and follow package directions.*

Cut cake horizontally to make 2 layers. (To split, mark side of cake with toothpicks and cut with long, thin serrated knife.)

Immediately before serving, top bottom layer with alternating scoops of half the sorbets and frozen yogurt. (Work quickly—it melts!) Sprinkle with half of the sliced fruits. Place top layer of cake firmly on the bottom layer, then top with rounded scoops of remaining frozen products and sprinkle with remaining fruit.

Drizzle sauce over all.

Makes 12 servings.

Per Serving: 143 Calories

Protein 2 gr.	Carb. 25 gr.
Fat 1 gr.	Cal. from fat 1%
Chol. 0 mg.	Sodium 190 mg.

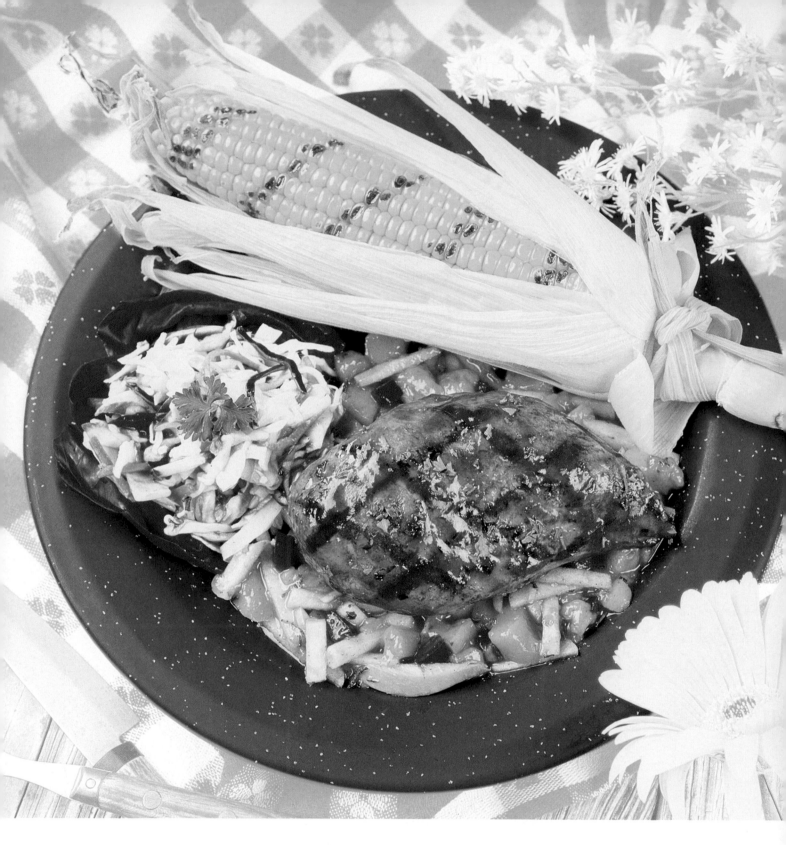

The days are long and lazy; it's time to enjoy the simple pleasure of cooking outdoors and eating relaxed meals on the deck. A down-home, all-American meal is in order: BBQ chicken, grilled corn on the cob and cole slaw make the perfect combination (pg. 196).

Fourth of July BBQ

Black Bean Dip
Fresh Vegetables
Creamy Herb Dip

Tortilla Chips
BBQ Breast of Chicken
Apple Chutney
Tricolor Coleslaw

Grilled Corn on the Cob
Peach Crisp
Summertime Fruit Pizza

Black Bean Dip

2 cans (15 oz. each) black beans, drained and rinsed
4 Tbsp. finely chopped canned or fresh jalapeño peppers
2 Tbsp. red wine vinegar
2 tsp. chili powder (or to taste)
1/2 tsp. creole seasoning
1/4 tsp. cumin
1 Tbsp. minced onion
1 tsp. minced garlic
1 Tbsp. chopped fresh parsley

- Serve with baked tortilla chips

Place in blender beans, peppers, vinegar, chili powder, seasoning and cumin. Blend until smooth. Transfer the mixture to a bowl.
Stir in onion, garlic and parsley.
Makes 12 servings, 1/3 cup each.

Per Serving: 117 Calories

Protein 8 gr.
Fat 0 gr.
Chol. 0 mg.

Carb. 21 gr.
Cal. from fat 0%
Sodium 68 mg.

Creamy Herb Dip

4 oz. light cream cheese, softened
1/4 cup nonfat sour cream
3 Tbsp. chopped fresh chives or scallions
1 Tbsp. chopped fresh dill
1/2 tsp. creole seasoning
1 tsp. Mrs. Dash seasoning
1 tsp. prepared horseradish

- Serve with fresh vegetables

Stir cream cheese into sour cream until smooth. Mix in chives, dill, seasonings and horseradish. Spoon into a small bowl. Wonderful with fresh vegetables.
Makes 4 servings, 1/4 cup each.

Per Serving: 24 Calories

Protein 4 gr.
Fat 0 gr.
Chol. 1 mg.

Carb. 1.5 gr.
Cal. from fat 0%
Sodium 147 mg.

Fourth of July BBQ (continued)

BBQ Breast of Chicken With Apple Chutney

½ cup Jamaican Marinade (pg. 57)
4 boneless, skinless chicken breast halves (1 lb.)
1 cup Citrus BBQ sauce (pg. 56)
1 ⅓ cups Apple Chutney

- Serve on a large platter over Apple Chutney.

Marinate chicken breasts in Jamaican Marinade for at least 1 hour. Grill, basting with Citrus BBQ sauce. Serve over Apple Chutney. Serves 4.

Per Serving: 252 Calories

Protein 28 gr.	Carb. 26 gr.
Fat 4 gr.	Cal. from fat 14%
Chol. 72 mg.	Sodium 410 mg.

Apple Chutney

1 Granny Smith apple, thinly julienned
1 cup Mango Chutney (pg. 62)

Mix together and refrigerate to blend flavors. Makes 4 servings, ⅓ cup each.

Per Serving: 47 Calories

Protein 0 gr.	Carb. 12 gr.
Fat 0 gr.	Cal. from fat 0%
Chol. 0 mg.	Sodium 272 mg.

Tricolor Coleslaw

2 cups red cabbage, shredded
2 cups green cabbage, shredded
1 cup carrots, grated
½ cup Citrus Vinaigrette (pg. 52)
2 Tbsp. chopped fresh herbs (cilantro, basil, rosemary, thyme)
½ tsp. creole seasoning
1 tsp. Mrs. Dash seasoning

In a large bowl, combine all ingredients, tossing well. Refrigerate until chilled. Serves 4.

Per Serving: 49 Calories

Protein 1 gr.	Carb. 8 gr.
Fat 1.5 gr.	Cal. from fat 29%
Chol. 1 mg.	Sodium 273 mg.

Grilled Corn on the Cob

4 ears of corn (with husks intact)

Carefully peel back husks, but do not detach. Remove silk; replace the husks back over the corn (leave a small bit exposed) and secure the top by pulling two pieces of husk to the front and tying into a bow-tie knot.
Microwave on high for 4 minutes.
Place exposed side of the corn on the grill, periodically turning for even cooking, until the ears are tender when pierced, about 8 minutes. Serves 4.

Per Serving: 83 Calories

Protein 2 gr.	Carb. 19 gr.
Fat 0 gr.	Cal. from fat 0%
Chol. 0 mg.	Sodium 13 mg.

entertain with style

Peach Crisp

10 medium peaches, sliced (or 4 cans,
   15½ oz. each, unsweetened
   sliced peaches)*
¾ cup golden raisins
3 Tbsp. canola oil
3 Tbsp. honey
1 cup old-fashioned oats, uncooked
½ tsp. allspice
1 tsp. cinnamon
¼ tsp. salt
⅓ cup whole-wheat pastry flour
2 Tbsp. walnuts
½ cup unsweetened white grape juice

*   may substitute sliced apples. Then bake
    for 40 to 45 minutes.

Preheat oven to 375 degrees.
Spread half of peaches in a large rectangular pan; top with raisins. Heat together the oil and honey. Add oats, allspice, cinnamon, salt, flour and walnuts. Crumble half of this mixture onto the peaches in the pan. Cover with remaining peaches and the rest of topping. Pour grape juice over the top.
Bake uncovered for 25 minutes.
Makes 12 servings.

Per Serving: 158 Calories

Protein 2.5 gr.	Carb. 28 gr.
Fat 4 gr.	Cal. from fat 23%
Chol. 0 mg.	Sodium 46 mg.

Summertime Fruit Pizza

1 burrito-sized fat-free flour tortilla
cinnamon
4 oz. fat-free cream cheese
¼ cup honey
1 tsp. vanilla
¼ cup fat-free ricotta cheese
3 kiwi, peeled and sliced
1 cup strawberries, sliced
1 peach or nectarine, sliced
¼ cup all-fruit apricot spread, warmed

Preheat oven to 375 degrees.
Spray a pizza pan with cooking spray. Place tortilla on pan; sprinkle lightly with cinnamon. Bake about 4 to 5 minutes until edges begin to lightly brown. Remove from oven and cool.
Beat together the cream cheese, honey and vanilla, then beat in the ricotta cheese till smooth. Spread the cheese mixture atop the cooled crust. Arrange the kiwi, strawberries and peaches on top, slightly overlapping. Chill in the refrigerator while preparing glaze.
Microwave the apricot spread in a small microwaveable bowl on high for 1 minute. Using a clean pastry brush, brush the glaze over the fruit. Chill 1 hour before serving.
Makes 6 servings.

Per Serving: 124 Calories

Protein 3 gr.	Carb. 28 gr.
Fat less than 1 gr.	Cal. from fat 3%
Chol. 0 mg.	Sodium 53 mg.

Recipe Index

Recipe Index (continued)

Recipe Index (continued)

Recipe Index (continued)

Recipe Index (continued)

Recipe Index (continued)

Subject Index

Tips Index

List of Charts and Tables

Metric Conversions

Metric Symbols

Celsius: C
liter: L
milliliter: mL
kilogram: kg

gram: g
centimeter: cm
millimeter: mm

Common Can/Package Sizes

VOLUME	MASS
4 oz. 114 mL	4 oz. 113 g
10 oz. 284 mL	5 oz. 142 g
14 oz. 398 mL	6 oz. 170 g
10 oz. 540 mL	7 $^3/_4$ oz. 220 g
28 oz. 796 mL	15 oz. 425 g

Oven Temperature Conversions

IMPERIAL	METRIC
250°F	120°C
275°F	140°C
300°F	150°C
325°F	160°C
350°F	180°C
375°F	190°C
400°F	200°C
425°F	220°C
450°F	230°C
500°F	260°C

Length

IMPERIAL	METRIC
$^1/_4$ inch	5 mm
$^1/_3$ inch	8 mm
$^1/_2$ inch	1 cm
$^3/_4$ inch	2 cm
1 inch	2.5 cm
2 inches	5 cm
4 inches	10 cm

Volume

IMPERIAL	METRIC
$^1/_4$ tsp.	1 mL
$^1/_2$ tsp.	2 mL
$^3/_4$ tsp.	4 mL
1 tsp.	5 mL
2 tsp.	10 mL
1 Tbsp.	15 mL
2 Tbsp.	25 mL
$^1/_4$ cup	50 mL
$^1/_3$ cup	75 mL
$^1/_2$ cup	125 mL
$^2/_3$ cup	150 mL
$^3/_4$ cup	175 mL
1 cup	250 mL
4 cups	1 L
5 cups	1.25 L

Mass (Weight)

IMPERIAL	METRIC
1 oz.	25 g
2 oz.	50 g
$^1/_4$ lb.	125 g
$^1/_2$ lb. (8 oz.)	250 g
1 lb.	500 g
2 lb.	1 kg
3 lb.	1.5 kg
5 lb.	2.2 kg
8 lb.	3.5 kg
10 lb.	4.5 kg
11 lb.	5 kg

This chart was developed by the Canadian Home Economics Association and the American Home Economics Committee. These guidelines were developed to simplify the conversion from Imperial measures to metric. The numbers have been rounded for convenience. When cooking from a recipe, work in the same system throughout the recipe; do not use a combination of the two.

Other Books by Pamela Smith, RD

- *The Energy Edge*—a groundbreaking approach to energized living. Filled with practical advice, this book will revolutionize your daily living.

- *The SMART Weigh Plan*—a five-point practical plan to health and fitness based on Strategic Eating and Drinking, Movement, Air, Rest and Treating your self well.

- *The Diet Trap*—How to win the fight against scale and excess weight—and live free of Diet Mania—to lose weight without losing yourself.

- *Eat Well—Live Well*—a guidebook helping thousands to eat for energy, peak performance, and disease prevention with a large recipe section.

- *Food for Life*—a strategic plan to feed your body, soul and spirit.

- *Healthy Expectations*—a pregnancy book with daily inspiration for your body, soul, and spirit. A large Q/A section is included with a proven strategy for overcoming morning sickness. A Journal edition is also available.

- *Alive and Well in the Fast Lane*—a fun book with the Ten Commandments of Good Nutrition. Perfect for teens and young adults.

- *Come Cook with Me*—a most extraordinary children's cookbook. Teach your children nutrition by teaching them how to cook.

For a free copy of
PAM'S LIVING WELL NEWSLETTER
and for ordering information, speaking and seminars
Contact 1.800.896.4010
Or visit www.pamsmith.com

Pamela Smith, R.D.

Pamela Smith, RD, nationally known nutritionist, energy coach, culinary consultant and best-selling author, designs delicious, healthy menus for hotels and restaurants worldwide such as Darden Restaurants and Hyatt Hotels and Resorts. She has coached professional and life athletes in winning plans from the NBA's Shaquille O'Neal, the PGA's Larry Nelson to Chuck Colson, as well as corporate giants such as Walt Disney World. She is the creator of *The Smart Weigh Lifestyle*® program through which thousands of people have found freedom from excess weight and ill health and have won back their energy for life.

Her best-selling books include *Eat Well Live Well*, *Food for Life*, *The Energy Edge* and *The Diet Trap*. She has hosted wellness shows for The Health Network, and her daily Living Well may be heard on radio stations nationwide. She has been featured on the *Today* Show, The TV Food Network, CNN News, MSNBC, Lifetime Television, *Focus on the Family*, *The 700 Club*, Larry Burket's *Money Matters*, *Janet Parshall's America*, *Life Today*, *Parent Talk* and many more.

Pam lives in Orlando, Florida with her husband, Larry, and their two daughters, Danielle and Nicole.